DETOX

Before You're

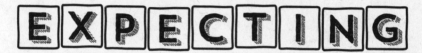

DETOX
Before You're
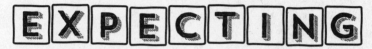
EXPECTING

A CLEANSING PROGRAM TO PREPARE
YOUR BODY FOR PREGNANCY

REA FREY

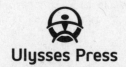

Ulysses Press

Published in the U.S. by
ULYSSES PRESS
P.O. Box 3440
Berkeley, CA 94703
www.ulyssespress.com

ISBN: 978-1-61243-402-5
Library of Congress Control Number 2014943014

Printed in Canada by Marquis Book Printing
10 9 8 7 6 5 4 3 2 1

Acquisitions Editor: Katherine Furman
Managing Editor: Claire Chun
Editor: Renee Rutledge
Proofreader: Lauren Harrison
Indexer: Sayre Van Young
Front cover design: Michelle Thompson
Interior design and layout: what!design @ whatweb.com
Cover illustrations: © Shanina/iStock.com

Distributed by Publishers Group West

NOTE TO READERS: This book has been written and published strictly for informational and educational purposes only. It is not intended to serve as medical advice or to be any form of medical treatment. You should always consult your physician before altering or changing any aspect of your medical treatment and/or undertaking a diet regimen, including the guidelines as described in this book. Do not stop or change any prescription medications without the guidance and advice of your physician. Any use of the information in this book is made on the reader's good judgment after consulting with his or her physician and is the reader's sole responsibility. This book is not intended to diagnose or treat any medical condition and is not a substitute for a physician.

To my pre-baby vagina:
I will always love you.

Contents

A Note to Readers

I know most of us want to know the secret to health. We want vibrant, radiant skin, a flat stomach, low cholesterol, a healthy heart, a stress-free life, and a million dollars. But here's the thing: There's no quick fix or easy answer to getting to the healthiest version of yourself. Period.

No author or expert (or even doctor) can tell you all the steps you need to take to get to your healthiest self. We are all different, which means we require different nutritional, emotional, physical, and mental needs. However, we can certainly gain the tools to make a positive change, which is what *Detox Before You're Expecting* aims to do.

Most of the books on the market today seem to regurgitate the same tired information. Eat whole foods! Stop eating processed crap! Exercise! Drink water! Reduce stress!

It's not always easy to implement these habits into our daily lives. We have deadlines to meet, bills to pay, and mouths to feed. There are too many foods to try, too many parties to attend, too many stressors, and too much temptation. And life is short, right? You might as well enjoy it!

While we can all live this mantra, the word "enjoyment" has taken on a vastly different meaning in today's world. Enjoyment often means sitting at a restaurant table, gorging ourselves on steaks and alcohol, then falling asleep in bed. What's so enjoyable about that? What happened to getting our enjoyment from activity, travel, and connecting with people (face-to-face and not via social media)? What happened to sending our children out to climb trees, make mud pies, or ride their bikes and telling them not to come home until dinner? What kind of enjoyment will your kids have? What world do you want to bring them into?

When you have children, everything does change. You have to reevaluate what you want your life to be and what you want theirs to be. And this can leave you with a lot of tough choices. But here's what's unacceptable: Passing down awful habits and nutritionally devoid foods to kids. Children should have the option to be introduced to healthy food. They should know what a vegetable is and why it's important to the body, and that yes, they can have candy on occasion, but that's the exception, not the rule. They should understand that eating foods in their natural state is always preferable to shoving their hands in a bag of chips. They should be involved in their choices—because learning about food is one of the best educations they can get.

But everyone feeds kids crap, right? Just look at any restaurant kids' menu. Look at the statistics. Look at how many kids are obese or sick or have adult illnesses, like diabetes. Their nutrition starts with your nutrition. In the beginning, it's up to you.

And because it's up to you, it starts with you. This book aims to help you clean out the junk from your system and press "reset" on your body before you conceive. Being pregnant is an amazing experience, but if you're not healthy, it can be unpleasant and put your baby at risk for unnecessary (i.e., preventable) health problems.

Be sensible with your choices. Find the parts of your life and diet that you can change and start to implement these tips, rules, and suggestions as you see fit.

We all slip up. We all fall off the wagon. We all love a good pizza or an ice-cold beer. But, as you'll soon learn, all of these behaviors can be changed or enjoyed moderately from time to time. You can still enjoy yourself. You can still be lenient and healthy. It's about changing the definition of what we think of as healthy. It's about starting a new chapter, or even a new page.

I hope you find something worthwhile within these pages. I hope this book inspires you to change even one habit and prepare yourself for parenthood in a more positive way.

I wish you the best of luck!

Happy parenting.

Introduction

Having been a vegetarian/vegan for over half my life, I'd returned to a meat-heavy diet in the years prior to getting pregnant. I was living in Chicago, which is heavy on environmental pollutants and smoking. Feeling sluggish and unhealthy, I decided to venture back to a completely plant-based diet. My husband decided to join me. Together, we began slowly eliminating and swapping our staple foods (you can read all about it in my book *Power Vegan: Plant-Fueled Nutrition for Maximum Health and Fitness*) with healthier, more nutrient-dense foods. We cleansed and felt our energy soar, unnecessary weight slough off, and stamina increase. After six months of plant-based eating, a detox, one colonic, and tons of water to flush my system, I got pregnant with our daughter Sophie. Thankfully, I was in the absolute best internal and external shape of my life.

Because of the proper steps I'd taken to get rid of the junk in my system, I knew what to eat, how to supplement, and what to feed my body and my growing baby. I swapped all of my makeup for natural choices and our household cleaning items for toxin-free, fragrance-free products. I learned that giving yourself an education on what you need and why you need it *before* you conceive is one of the biggest gifts you can give yourself, rather than jumping in blind.

Bun in the Oven

Getting pregnant: There is no scarier or exciting time. Almost as soon as you see that plus sign staring back at you, the questions begin. What doctor should I see? Do I want a midwife? How am I going to afford this? Will the baby be healthy? Am I ever going to sleep again? (No, you're not.)

Before you lose yourself in a sea of baby books or opinionated mothers who will tell you how to do things *their* way, your prime focus should be making your pregnancy easier, happier, and stress-free: *getting healthy before you conceive.* Though health means many different things to everyone (especially in today's overly saturated health and wellness market), we all want to be healthy and stay that way. But first, you must define what health means to you.

What if you could get your body to a clean slate before you conceive? Ensuring that you are the healthiest version of yourself will promote an easier pregnancy and delivery. According to the USDA article "The Importance of Nutrition in Pregnancy for Lifelong Health," mothers who are fit and healthy have lower blood pressure, fewer issues during pregnancy, and an easier labor, delivery, and recovery. Many of these mothers are able to handle natural births with no medical interventions, and their babies are usually healthier. While there are always unforeseen "issues" in delivery (my 52-hour labor, for one), preparing yourself pre-pregnancy to handle almost anything thrown your way helps ready you mentally as well as physically for the screaming, lack of sleep, and intense hormonal highs and lows you will now experience for the rest of your life. (P.S. Having a baby makes you much more honest. And sarcastic.)

The process of removing toxins from the body can happen in innumerable ways. Ask around, and most likely, someone has a story of how they cleansed. Superfood smoothies, juice cleanses, full-body organ cleanses, pills, retreats, meditations, fasts... Name an issue, a detox method exists. But what works best for some people can seem daunting and expensive to others.

Case in point: Despite being a health and fitness professional, the first time I tried a juice cleanse, I made it about five hours before I broke down and stuffed my face with sprouted toast, almond butter, and copious amounts of coffee. I love food that much. The idea of deprivation has never worked for me. If I know I will have to go three days without food, I will find a way to have it. I will research every angle that contends juice cleanses are bad for you and justify my inability to cleanse myself. This is why a whole-foods cleanse like the one I recommend in this book makes sense to so many people. While you omit the bad "trigger" foods, you can swap them with good, nutritious options that won't leave you deprived and will make you feel fantastic. No second and third trips to the coffee pot—guaranteed.

If you are ready to conceive (or are already pregnant and want to get healthy), you might not have time to research all the different routes to take (or have the patience for a juice cleanse). Which has brought you here, to me.

I have always been a food lover, but I have also been educated in nutrition, health, wellness, and all facets of whole-foods, plant-based living for the past fifteen years. I think the safest way to detoxify the body is through the elimination and reintroduction of certain foods. While fasts and juice cleanses may be absolutely vital to those patients dealing with severe health issues, this book is a gentle-cleansing program meant to help a woman get to the healthiest version of herself—pre-pregnancy. But you have to do the work.

Getting a handle on what your body does and doesn't like is incredibly important when thinking about carrying a baby. What your body is asked to do—create a human that will sap your body of vital nutrients and minerals and steal your soul for the next eighteen years—is an exhausting, miraculous task. Period.

This is where *Detox Before You're Expecting* comes in. I will take you step-by-step through detoxifying the natural way with whole, plant-based foods, healthy habits, and tried-and-true methods.

Warning: While many people experience weight loss and increased energy with detoxing, this is neither a diet nor a "fad." It's simply eliminating nutritional stress, toxins, and allergens and allowing your body to cleanse itself so you can actually process nutrients the way nature intended: effortlessly.

Take it from someone in the throes of parenthood (terrible two's, be gone!), the time before you conceive is golden. Sleep until you can't sleep anymore, drink plenty of water, eat good, quality food, have sex until your body parts fall off, and realize that how healthy you are before you conceive (this goes for your partner as well) plays dramatically in your pregnancy experience and post-birth recovery.

Because I was healthy pre-pregnancy, during pregnancy, and post-pregnancy, we have had no major issues. My daughter enjoys healthy, nutritious food. We've had no countless trips to the doctor's office. No missing bowel movements, strange rashes, incessant colds, or flus. No food allergies. No labored breathing. We started her with a good base (breast milk) and ventured into offering whole foods. We are now letting her gravitate toward food that she is interested in as she grows. Laying this healthy foundation can be one of the most important things you ever do. What better place to start than with yourself?

For better or worse, becoming a parent changes you, humbles you, scares you, and gives you something entirely outside of yourself worth living for.

Now, it's time to give your child (or future child) the same gift back: a healthy parent.

CHAPTER ONE

What Is Detoxification and Why Do We Need It?

Detoxification is not a new phenomenon. Whether for spiritual cleansing, natural medicine, or even colonic irrigation, the process of detoxifying the body, spirit, and mind has been around for centuries. Explains Johnny Cooke, MS, RTSm, MATm, licensed occupational therapist and cofounder of Precision Human Performance:

> Detoxification, or detox, refers to the removal or extraction of substances carrying potential long- or short-term risks to the biological makeup of a living organism. These substances are minimized by pathways the body already has in place.

Our bodies contain toxins from bacteria, fungus, parasites, chemicals, and other substances. These toxins can come from the environment, our lifestyle choices, and the foods and beverages we consume. Once the toxins have been produced, we have systems in place to limit and excrete them.

None of what we consume or produce that carries the risk of damage to us is unknown to the internal environment. There's nothing that the body isn't prepared for—it has steps in place to defend itself. It's a question of whether the body becomes overwhelmed.

It's vital to remember that it's much more about *how much* we consume than *what* we consume, as we've been previously taught.

For example, if I consume carcinogens every day in small enough doses that my body can take care of as a single "event," I won't reap as many negative effects as I would if I were to consume large, ongoing doses. It's when these larger doses of toxins become a constant event that they manifest as a problem.

Remember, it's not the toxin or carcinogen we take in that's the real culprit—it's our body's *response* to it that becomes dangerous.

Our bodies don't think long-term. The body *is* cause and effect, which proves it is smarter than we give it credit for. But we get in our own way. We decrease the body's efficiency through the way we eat, the toxins we consume, and the lifestyles we lead.

When we detoxify, we literally remove toxins from the system. Johnny explains:

> There is substantial evidence that human physiology is equipped with every necessary facet to remove damaging substances from the body. The goal of detox strategies is to provide the window of opportunity for metabolism to

do its job (by reducing foreign ingestion) and to bolster efficiency through the appropriate dosages of metabolic stress in the form of exercise.

While exercise does cause metabolic stress and damage, if done in the appropriate dosages, it's the damage that starts the processes that *repair* the body. If you don't exercise or restrict calories enough (i.e., you overeat and intermittently reduce caloric intake), you get stealth damage (flying-under-the-radar damage). This type of damage happens constantly, but not at high enough levels to signal an alarm. Nothing ever happens (internally) to stop it. And then bam! When you're fifty, you have a heart attack. Or you get cancer. Or you just drop dead.

If you don't overeat or consume toxic chemicals (and if you practice appropriate levels of physical exertion), the body is constantly in a state of detox. Our bodies are *designed* to get rid of toxins, but we very rarely give our bodies that opportunity. As babies, we start with a somewhat clean slate (though we are only as healthy as our parents allow) and just add and add and add to the toxic buildup. Think about the duration of our lives. From the first day to now, what have we consumed and ingested? From antibiotics and other prescription medications, drugs, alcohol, additives, chemicals, hormones, preservatives, environmental toxins, and processed foods to relationship and professional stressors, we consume and consume. Now, have you ever skipped a bowel movement? Or a workout? Where do you think all that you accumulate goes?

Our bodies aim to get rid of the "bad stuff," but when we slow them down so much by clogging them up, we get into trouble. Not eliminating properly, eating the wrong foods, gaining weight, staying sedentary, using products made with chemicals, breathing in environmental toxins—these are all factors that prevent natural detoxification and optimal health.

We are so focused on treatment-based thinking (from bringing down a fever to curing a headache, we look for ways to fix the problem) that we miss the opportunity for *causative* thinking. Why is that rash there? Why have I not had a bowel movement in two days? Why do I get consistent headaches? Why am I tired all the time? Trying to get to the root of the issue instead of medicating the symptoms is an important part of healing your mind and body: This is where detoxification comes into play.

We can learn to detoxify naturally. All we have to do is get out of the way of the process. While we are all so focused on detoxing, Johnny explains that we need to stop detoxing. Instead, we need to stop "toxifying" our systems. So, focus on what you can do to eliminate toxins in the body. An immediate way to start? Stop with the overconsumption of calories, lack of exercise, and consumption of dangerous toxins.

Detoxification takes on many forms (fasts, herbal cleanses, elimination diet, juicing, etc.), but the ultimate purpose is the same: to reach optimal health. While these tactics have been around for quite some time, the safest and most effective way to detoxify the system is through whole-foods cleansing. This type of cleansing gives you adequate control of what goes into your body, provides essential nutrients and minerals, and can be maintained for a lifetime. It is a long-term health solution, not a quick diet fix.

In *Staying Healthy with Nutrition*, Dr. Elson Haas, MD, discusses how cleansing can increase chances of conception, balance hormones, flush out toxins, banish food intolerances, and help manage future cravings. We can contribute to this cleansing by monitoring what we eat and don't eat and making permanent lifestyle changes.

Food Fight

Health is not a single event. It's a culmination of lifelong habits, from dietary choices to the way we handle stress at work. Food is merely one component of the overall picture, but it can be the hardest one to "nail" in terms of finding a healthy middle ground. Food—something we must partake in every single day, multiple times per day just to survive—can make or break a person's threshold for other pollutants. The stronger your immune system, the easier it is to kick other pollutants and illnesses from your body, which is why detoxifying your body is so important.

"Food can hurt us or heal us, and given what's happening to us on the current SAD (standard American diet), it is, frankly, now killing us. That SAD is full of foods that are toxic to our bodies and minds because it is a diet comprised of mostly refined, overly processed, and mass-manufactured food," Alex Jamieson writes in *The Great American Detox Diet*. The propensity to be overweight is another reason for Americans to cleanse. According to the Centers for Disease Control and Prevention, more than 35 percent of the American population is obese.

Maybe you're not obese. Then, you're probably healthy, right? Wrong. It's not being overweight that's unhealthy—it's the *process* of gaining weight that's unhealthy. Johnny Cooke explains:

> The amount of food that you eat, regardless of the nourishment within it, is as bad as eating the wrong foods. Overeating will give you cancer and kill you. You can actually maintain your calories, exercise, and be healthy when you're slightly overweight, versus someone who grossly overeats and is in a constant state of gaining and losing weight. This is where the danger happens. This is but one indicator that things are going

south. But weight is only *one* indicator among countless indicators of what's going on in and outside our bodies.

Okay, so what do we do? The thought of change can be scary, especially when it comes to food or habits. We are a ritualistic society. We relate the food we eat to the good times we have. The imminent fear remains that if we start eating healthy food, we won't be spontaneous when it comes to frequenting the restaurants we enjoy. Eating good food goes hand in hand with being social. What happens when we're eating better, while the whole world drowns in decadent fare?

This is where you must find the balance. Finding restaurants that offer healthier options and enjoying social outings for reasons beyond food are good first steps in changing your mindset. You can still enjoy the things you love and be healthy. If we start thinking about the consequences of what we eat and how often we eat it, we might start thinking a bit differently in terms of what we're "entitled" to. Jeffrey A. Morrison, MD, writes in *Cleanse Your Body, Clear Your Mind*:

> After prolonged exposure to a toxic diet, the digestive tract eventually loses the good bacteria necessary to digest and help absorb nutrients properly. Bad bacteria or yeast begin to colonize in the colon. The change causes food to ferment in the intestines, creating gas and bloating. Worse, the new bacteria and yeast aren't recognized by the immune system, 70 percent of which is located in the digestive tract. Instead, the bacteria and yeast are considered foreign, stimulating an immune system response and causing inflammation in the digestive tract, which leads to a breakdown in the normal structure of the intestines.

This inflammation, which allows incompletely digested food to be absorbed, can lead to what we call leaky gut syndrome. If you suffer from low-grade fevers or inconsistent gut pain that doesn't make sense, leaky gut syndrome could be to blame. Because the body works so hard to regulate itself, the immune system is constantly working and can therefore burn out.

"Often the foods you most frequently eat will become the most toxic to your system," Morrison writes. Why? Because our bodies can develop food sensitivities and allergies from the foods we most commonly consume. If you are eating the trigger foods (wheat, dairy, soy, eggs, etc.) that are usually genetically modified or pumped with hormones or pesticides, your body will do whatever it can to expel these toxins. But, after a while, it can't.

It's no surprise that so many food sensitivities and allergies have cropped up. Everywhere you go, you hear about dairy-, gluten-, meat-, egg-, and soy-free foods. Twenty years ago, it seemed that people weren't allergic to as many things. In the CNN article "Why Are Food Allergies on the Rise?" Elizabeth Landau writes, "The number of kids with food allergies went up 18 percent from 1997 to 2007, according to the US Centers for Disease Control and Prevention. About 3 million children younger than 18 had a food or digestive allergy in 2007." The speculations about food allergies run rampant, from our children not having enough of the right gut bacteria to not being exposed to nuts and shellfish at an early enough age, to the standard American diet, to our environments being too stripped of germs to elicit the proper immune response.

Unsafe food practices and overproduction are also to blame. Traditionally, animals weren't pumped full of hormones and antibiotics. We weren't churning out cheap crops, spraying them with horrible pesticides (remember that the whole point of pesticides is to kill things!), and injecting corn, soy, and wheat into every food possible. The growth and manufacturing practices are different, which makes the product different, which makes consumption different. In spending so much time trying to break down food it doesn't recognize, the body isn't given the chance to function properly.

This is why detoxification, *especially* in this day and age, is so needed.

Confused about which ingredients are okay and which aren't? Just use common sense. If you aren't sure or can't pronounce an ingredient, move on to another product. Start with this list and take inventory of the foods you purchase or consume.

The Crap List

Additives/Emulsifiers/Preservatives

- Acetylated esters of mono and diglycerides
- Artificial colors
- Artificial flavors (and artificially flavored drinks, packaged goods, etc.)
- Autolyzed proteins
- Benzoates
- Bleached flour
- Bromated flour
- Brominated vegetable oil (BVO)
- Caffeine
- Canola oil (rapeseed oil)
- Carmine
- Casein
- Certified colors
- Corn (modified cornstarch, dextrose, maltodextrin, corn oil, corn syrup, and even fresh corn)
- Diacetyl tartaric and fatty acid esters of mono and diglycerides (DATEM)
- Dimethylpolysiloxane
- Enriched wheat
- Ethoxyquin
- Ethyl vanillin
- FD&C colors
- Hexa-, hepta-, and octa-esters of sucrose
- High-fructose corn syrup
- Hydrogenated fats
- Hydrolyzed vegetable protein
- Lactylated esters of mono and diglycerides
- Methylparaben
- Microparticularized whey protein–derived fat substitute
- Monosodium glutamate (MSG)

- Nitrates/nitrites
- Olestra
- Partially hydrogenated oil
- Polydextrose
- Polysorbate 80
- Potassium benzoate
- Potassium bromate
- Potassium sorbate
- Propionates
- Propyl gallate
- Propylparaben
- Sorbic acid
- Soy lecithin
- Sulfites
- Tertiary butylhydroquinone (TBHQ)
- Tetrasodium EDTA
- Vanillin
- Yeast extract

Chemicals/Compounds

- Acrylamides
- Ammonium chloride
- Azodicarbonamide
- Benzoyl peroxide
- Bisphenol A (BPA)
- Butylated hydroxyanisole (BHA)
- Butylated hydroxytoluene (BHT)
- Calcium bromate
- Calcium disodium ethylenediaminetetraacetic acid (EDTA)
- Calcium peroxide
- Calcium propionate
- Calcium saccharin
- Calcium sorbate
- Calcium stearoyl-2-lactylate
- Caprocaprylobehenin
- Cysteine (L-cysteine)
- Dioctyl sodium sulfosuccinate (DSS)
- Disodium calcium EDTA
- Disodium dihydrogen EDTA
- Disodium guanylate (GMP)
- Disodium inosinate (IMP)
- EDTA
- Ethylene oxide
- Hydrochloride
- Methyl silicon
- Phosphoric acid
- Propylene glycol
- Sodium
- Sodium aluminum sulfate
- Sodium benzoate
- Sodium diacetate
- Sodium glutamate
- Sodium nitrate/nitrite
- Sodium propionate
- Sodium stearoyl-2-lactylate

Sweeteners

- Acesulfame-K (acesulfame potassium)
- Aspartame
- Cyclamates
- Saccharin
- Sucralose
- Sucroglycerides
- Sucrose polyester
- Sugar

Other

- Factory-farmed meat
- Foie gras
- Genetically Modified Organisms (GMOs)
- Homogenized milk
- Hydrogenated fats
- Imitation foods
- Irradiated foods
- Lead-soldered cans
- Solvent extracted oils, such as soybean oil, corn oil, or canola oil (except grapeseed oil)
- Soy (a GMO, as appearing in processed foods)
- Soy protein
- Textured vegetable protein

Watch What (and How Much) You Eat—Even the Good Stuff

Right before my daughter turned two, I had slipped back into some familiar habits: organic peanut butter, coconut oil with almost every meal, cacao, black beans, flaxseeds, cashews, etc. I ate healthy food, but a lot of it, and had gotten into a rut with eating the same foods almost daily. I began experiencing strange symptoms. For a few months, on various occasions, I developed low-grade fevers out of nowhere and intense gastrointestinal problems. It didn't seem like a regular virus, and I couldn't pinpoint the issue. Taking all of my beloved foods with me to my holistic practitioner, we tested them on his handy electrodermal analysis machine, which can read your body's frequency in relation to the foods you eat or the supplements you take. To best explain it: If something registers high on the scale, it is taxing to your body. Coffee would be a prime example, attacking the adrenals and making your body work harder than it has to. If a food or supplement registers low, your body literally cannot digest that food and it is doing more harm than good.

Because we live in a world where we lump all the "healthy" foods in one box and all the "unhealthy" foods in another, we have come to believe that if we eat something healthy, we can indulge in it as much as we want to. You can't possibly eat too many seeds, or nuts, or grains, right? Wrong.

As we went through the bag of foods I ate the most often, I discovered that flax, black beans, peanut butter, cacao, cashews, and my beloved coconut oil were detrimental to my body. My body was struggling so hard to digest things it didn't want and couldn't adequately break down. I was shocked.

I found it ironic that my body didn't want most of the items that had been deemed "healthy." Was it the food or the *frequency* and *amounts* that I was eating them? I started making those swaps and reductions and haven't had a single issue since. Some will say it's a coincidence and others will wonder if I have to stay away from those foods forever.

The frequency and amounts of foods we eat are more important than what we are eating. Do you mostly eat the same foods every day? If you eat the same ingredients every single day, your body will get used to that food and can even start to become "immune" to it over time. You stop reaping the benefits as your body struggles to find varied nutrition elsewhere.

Does this mean that if you eat a bowl of oatmeal every single day, your body will stop absorbing the nutrients? No. But it will certainly miss out on other nutrients that come from different ingredients. Because the bulk of our diets usually doesn't stem from fresh, whole, unprocessed foods, our bodies adapt to what we are eating and crave real nutritional content—not just calories. If you continue to eat the same foods every single day without variation, you are essentially starving your body of nutritional variety.

So not varying our diets is one of the first places we start to get in trouble, especially if yours is nutrient-deprived. If all you ever eat for lunch is chicken and a salad, your body misses out on other vital nutrients. This is why a "meat and potatoes" diet, as many of us are brought up on, offers little nutrition, other than protein. It's important to ingest those ever-important micronutrients often found in plant-based food.

The amount of what we eat is the secondary component. Too much of anything eaten over and over and over again can have a negative effect on your body. So, even if someone tells you to gorge on coconut oil and kale, make sure you eat everything, even the good stuff, in moderation. The volume of what we eat (which we will soon discuss) is just as important as *what* we eat.

The Other Toxins

Besides those found in food, we contend with other toxins on an almost-daily basis. What about those toxins we can't see? What about the environmental pollutants, mold, and heavy metals? You can clean up your diet, but if you continue to handle toxic substances, especially when pregnant or post-delivery, you will continually expose yourself and your child to these triggers that will affect your health.

Look out for these dangerous toxins found in everyday products, from household cleaners, cosmetics, and body washes to shampoos and conditioners, kids' toys, toothpaste, and paint:

- Acrylamide
- Alachlor
- Arsenic
- Asbestos
- Atrazine
- Barium
- Benzene
- Benzophenone-3, or oxybenzone
- Beryllium

- Bisphenol A (BPA)
- Boric acid
- Bromate
- Butyl-hydroxyanisole (BHA)
- Cadmium
- Carbon monoxide
- Catechol
- Chlorine
- Chlorite
- Chromium
- Copper
- Cryptosporidium
- Cyanide
- Dalapon
- Dibutyl phthalate (DBP)
- Dinoseb
- Dioxin
- Ethyl paraben
- Ethylbenzene
- Ethylene dibromide
- Ethylene oxide
- Fire retardants
- Fluoride
- Genetically modified organisms (GMOs)
- Giardia lamblia
- Ground-level ozone
- Hormones (added to food supply)
- Lead
- Legionella
- Lindane
- Mercury
- Mold
- Nitrate
- Nitrite
- Nitrogen dioxide
- Particulate matter
- Pentachlorophenol
- Pesticides (organophosphates, carbamate, organochlorine, DEET, fluoride)
- Petrolatum
- Plasticizers (phthalates and bisphenol A)
- Polychlorinated biphenyls (PCBs)
- Preservatives
- Propylparaben
- Selenium
- Styrene
- Sulfur dioxide
- Thallium
- Trichloroethylene (TCE)
- Volatile organic compounds (VOCs)

This can seem like a daunting and exhaustive list. After all, our bodies can adapt to many of these pollutants because they just can't be avoided. Take baby steps to change one thing at a time for drastically improved health effects.

Detoxification Programs

Before partaking in any sort of detoxification program, it's imperative to get your blood work done to make sure there are no underlying issues that might require medical attention. If you are someone who wants to eat according to your blood type, there are many resources out there that can help you along the way.

Many doctors can even test for mercury, mold, and food sensitivities to see if you might be allergic to any environmental or indoor pollutants or have food-related allergies or sensitivities. Going into pregnancy and this cleanse with as much information about yourself as possible will make all the difference in how successful you are. Once you have been cleared, it's good to start slowly so as not to completely shock the system.

For your whole-foods cleanse, we will start with the eight most common food triggers: dairy, caffeine, alcohol, meat, sugar, peanuts, soy, and wheat, weaning you off slowly and incorporating healthier, whole foods into your diet to get you ready for a healthy pregnancy. Mercury will also be discussed, since mercury levels in fish have become incredibly high, and the toxicity of fish does not often outweigh the benefits of consumption. Mercury-free supplements will be recommended in place of most types of mercury-laden fish, especially while cleansing or pregnant.

Now that you know what detoxification is and why we need to cleanse the body, what kinds of detoxification programs exist, and what are the risks and benefits of each?

Fasting

Fasting has been around for centuries. Many cultures practice fasting as a way to heal, foster discipline, or get closer to God.

Intermittent fasting, or intermittent caloric deficit, is less prevalent in our society. There's often a misunderstanding of the definition of the term "fasting." As Johnny Cooke explains:

> It is important to note that "fasting" is defined by a reduction in calories by roughly 25 percent below the baseline caloric intake of an individual. The "fasting" period would be three to five days and reduce to that only every fourteen to twenty-one days.

This is a loose guideline for intermittent fasting. So fasting doesn't necessarily mean no food—it's a completely strategic and scientific endeavor that should always be monitored by a seasoned professional.

BENEFITS: Intermittent fasting can give the digestive system time to rest, repair, and heal. In fact, we are not going to reap health unless we incorporate intermittent fasting, which means only reducing our calories by 25 percent for a few days. We are so used to eating every few hours that giving the body a break to repair and eliminate waste can be beneficial for our digestive systems. Usually, these fasts occur during a certain part of the day or week, and some food and water are incorporated to prevent negative side effects. Johnny Cooke explains, "Fasting can also be critical to favorable biochemical processes and allows activation of important post-glycogen-depletion metabolic processes."

What does this mean? There are specific enzymes that can only become active when you are depleted of glycogen for a sustained period of time. It takes roughly 24 to 36 hours to get to your resting blood glucose levels. You need to run a deficit for at least that period of time before you can potentially say that you are depleted of glycogen. Why is this important? "If you have a surplus of glycogen, you can't run a deficit, and you won't reap the health benefits that come with that depletion," Johnny states. "There are disease-fighting enzymes that are produced in this post-glycogen state. It has a favorable effect on body composition. You minimize the stress response of having to metabolize the glucose."

It's important to remember that everything we consume becomes glucose. When you're depleted of glycogen (because you've exercised and restricted calories or you've restricted calories for a long enough period of time), you ease the load of having to metabolize glucose and its byproducts that can be damaging in high enough doses.

Fasting can also support positive body composition by reducing caloric adaption when used intermittently. "While drastic fasting or calorie reduction (that results in a deficit) can have *some* benefits, fasting should never be sustained for longer than 48 hours and never ever while pregnant," Johnny cautions. This is why intermittent caloric deficit can be such a good way to detoxify the body effortlessly and often without cutting out food.

RISKS: Whenever you deny the body food, you prohibit the absorption and digestion of vital nutrients and minerals. The fat storage mechanism kicks in, and the body tries to preserve what it has to survive. If extended, this can become dangerous. The body will weaken from lack of energy and processes can slow down, especially if not properly hydrated. Fasting can lead to extreme dehydration, fatigue, and loss of mental clarity and should only be done under supervision of a professional. Besides nutrient insufficiencies or deficiencies, overuse and abuse of the strategy are common and can lead to negative side effects.

Juicing

The juicing craze has many pros and cons. It consists simply of extracting the juices from whole fruits and veggies and then consuming the juices. The thought process behind juicing is if the fiber is stripped, you are giving the digestive system a break and delivering vitamins and minerals directly to the bloodstream.

BENEFITS: Juicing has been proven to cure ailments, shed weight, and increase vitality and health. Because of its convenient and concentrated delivery system for nutrients and phytocompounds, it can be an obvious choice for those who want to cleanse the body. It's also an easy way to get your greens in if you have an aversion to plant-based foods. According to Betsy Reed, holistic health business consultant:

> If done with an outcome or specific goal in mind, short-term juicing (less than five days) of organic herbs, fruits, and vegetables puts all of the key nutrients directly into your body, without making your body do the work of digestion. That's why juicing is a huge part of the healing process: It cleanses, nourishes, and eliminates—all without making extra work for your body, so it can truly heal.

For the most benefits, juice should always be consumed on an empty stomach and not mixed with other foods.

RISKS: Juice fasts tend to be high in sugar, lack fiber, and have a high caloric content. Depending on the ingredients, you can have a high caloric content with low food bulk, which can lead to an overconsumption of overall calories. There's also a potential for hypervitaminosis (high storage level of vitamins, which can lead to toxic symptoms) for some individuals. The weight most people lose while juicing is water and will be regained once solid food is consumed. Betsy explains:

> Obsessive juicing for pure weight loss can be damaging. Cleanses are meant to be done one to two times per year as a "reset," or a way to stave off disease. When done regularly, juice cleanses can actually have the opposite

effect of healing and slow metabolism and disrupt the healthy work of the body doing its job of digestion.

Organic produce is always preferred, as conventional fruits and veggies that contain pesticides are delivered directly to the blood without any scrubbing fiber to help eliminate waste (which can hinder the healing process). Many popular juice and smoothie chains offer juices with conventional produce, which should be avoided, especially if doing a juice cleanse prior to pregnancy. Always ask if the juices are made with organic produce.

Herbal Cleanses

Herbal cleanses, or "boxed" cleanses, as they are sometimes referred to, can be helpful when it comes to organ and heavy-metal detoxification. Herbs have been around for centuries and can be vital in helping rid the body of toxins. However, many people do not follow the other rules when taking these cleanses and will not completely eliminate sugar, alcohol, caffeine, processed foods, medications, etc. Many feel there are not enough benefits in order to safely cleanse.

BENEFITS: Many people thrive with herbal cleanses and specialty detoxes, reporting improved sleep, better digestion, clearer skin, and healthier organs. It can be a great maintenance program for those who need "tune-ups" every now and then. Just as with a juice cleanse, only the purest essential oils and best organic herbs should be used.

RISKS: Some people are allergic to herbs, but do not know they are allergic until after consuming them. Also, herbs can interfere with certain prescribed medications, so it's vital to check with your doctor to see about possible contraindications. Herbal cleanses can also draw heavy metals into the bloodstream (or placenta, if pregnant). There can be cardiac concerns for some patients as well. Many herbal cleanses are poorly researched in biochemistry and metabolic functions and therefore do not have enough substantial scientific research to support them. If you ever purchase herbal cleanses, always look for those made in the United States, as many herbal supplements made in China and India are infiltrated with high levels of pesticides and heavy metals.

Whole-Foods Program

A whole-foods detoxification program can be a balanced program in which the person can experiment with what foods feel best for his or her diet. As Betsy states:

> Our body's job is to heal, digest, and sleep. Utilizing a combination of juice or smoothie in the morning, followed by fresh whole foods for the rest of the day permits the body to heal and do what it is designed to do. A primarily plant-based diet (heavy on greens) is easily digestible and creates very little trauma to the body.

Think of fresh, whole foods as "clean" foods; foods in their natural state that have not been altered or processed.

BENEFITS: By eliminating trigger foods and incorporating healthier fare into the diet, one can experience numerous benefits, which include increased energy, improved bowel function, weight loss, lower blood pressure, absence of allergies and colds, lower cholesterol, clear skin, and improved sex drive. Because there's an appropriate delivery system for nutrients and phytocompounds, there's a lower risk of hyper consumption of certain nutrients (i.e., it's more balanced and not as concentrated, as in juicing). There's minimal risk with whole-foods detoxing, as you're "getting out of your own way" to let the detox happen. You are also receiving bulk nutrition, fiber, and roughage to help the body eliminate toxins and heal with food—not the lack of it.

RISKS: Because you are not completely eliminating all food, it's sometimes hard to reach a "clean" slate without fasting, doing colonics, or juicing beforehand. What one person deems as a "healthy" whole-foods cleanse can still include processed foods or allergen-rich foods if they are not aware of what should be consumed or avoided. There's also potential not to reach adequate requirements of all macronutrients if you are on a strict, plant-based, Atkins, paleo, or other limiting diet without proper knowledge of where to get all of your macro and micronutrients. Overconsuming calories is a danger, even with those so-called "good" foods. Calories are still calories and will be stored as fat if you are eating more than you are moving or your base metabolic rate is burning.

Aiding Your Detox

It's important to note that with any of these cleanses, there are other things you can do to aid your detox. From colonics/enemas, skin scrubs, and Epsom salt baths to massages, hot yoga, exercise, and stress relief, detoxifying both the mind and body take more than just picking up a piece of celery.

It's important to analyze the areas of your life outside of your diet that might need some help. Ask yourself:

AM I HAPPY IN MY JOB? If not, where does most of the stress stem from? Is it preventable stress (e.g., not being organized) or is it linked to money (e.g., not getting paid what you're worth)?

AM I HAPPY IN MY RELATIONSHIP? Look at what is fixable, such as bad habits or communication, and what's not, such as wanting a partner to be completely different to match your specific needs.

AM I SOCIALLY FULFILLED? Do you have a good support network of friends and family? Do you find yourself feeling lonely?

Study the areas in your life that might need a proper detox, then take the adequate steps to eliminate stress and bolster confidence. Use detoxifying your body as the first step to a calmer, healthier, more productive life.

The Skinny

Do your research and experiment with different cleanses that feel right to you and address your specific symptoms. For some, doing a short juice detox before entering into a whole-foods detox may be just as beneficial as exploring colonics or other ways to detoxify the body.

While it's vital to do your research and see which cleanse will best benefit you before pregnancy, the whole-foods cleanse is an ideal program for immediate, *lasting* results. On the whole-foods detoxification program outlined in this book for beginner to advanced levels, you will stay satiated while cutting out the junk in your diet.

The focus of this program is on replacing unhealthy foods with whole foods, while paying attention to the amount you're eating—not just what you're eating. This will offer a safe and effective way of naturally detoxifying the body. Through identifying culprit foods, as well as environmental and lifestyle factors, you can address specific *daily* issues or preferences and see how your body reacts with safe food elimination and healthy swaps.

This is not a rigid program. You do not have to follow every single food option or suggestion or meal plan. There are no strictly set serving sizes or portions, because the entire point of this cleanse is to tune in to see what *your* body wants and needs. We all have different activity levels and lifestyles, which much be taken into account.

On this program, you will do the work, just as you will do the work when you are pregnant.

In addition to replacing processed foods with healthier foods, there is an option to toggle calories. For those who count calories or want a more definitive way to track your progress, you will toggle calories on certain days to give your body a chance to "reset" itself and detoxify naturally while losing weight. Not interested? Not to worry.

The choices you make through this book and beyond are yours and yours alone.

That's why this program is catered to *personal* decisions, preferences, and choices that will not only prepare you for pregnancy but will sustain you for the rest of your life.

CHAPTER TWO

Why Whole-Foods Detoxing?

Our bodies are made to eat "real" food. What's real food? Whole foods, or foods that come from the ground and are in their most natural state. Think about that definition and compare it to what you eat. What percentage of your diet is composed of truly whole foods that haven't been altered into something packaged, processed, or cooked at high temperatures? Think about that percentage on a daily, weekly, and yearly basis, and then span decades. Think about, on average, how much food you ingest every day as compared to how much you eliminate. Now, think about the amount of days you've ever gone in your life without eliminating after every meal (which would mean three to five times per day). Think about food still hanging out in your gut, manifesting in disease or weight gain. Think about the prescription (or recreational) drugs you've taken, alcohol consumed, pollutants inhaled, and chemicals worn on your clothes, let alone the ones that lurk in your products, paint, furniture, and even your technology. Think you might need a little help in cleaning out your system? Most of us do.

But why should we opt for a whole-foods detoxification program? It's not a "quick" fix, right? Wouldn't it be better to just juice or fast instead? I always recommend that people focus on elimination first. Whole foods contain fiber, the secret weapon for flushing toxins from our systems.

As an added benefit, whole-foods detoxification can occur year-round and be altered to fit exercise needs, lifestyle changes, or even allergies (both food and environmental). With a revised grocery list and a willingness to make a few healthy changes, the results with how you look and feel can be immediate.

Whole foods deliver the most vital nutrients to our systems and supply us with the energy and means to go about our day. Whole foods are made to be eaten; though we have gotten away from eating foods that come from the ground and are in their most natural state since the invention of processed food, it's easy to turn back to nature and opt for food that's as close to its natural state as possible.

When we eat whole foods, we provide the body with instant energy. Foods such as fruits and vegetables are easy to digest. They don't steal energy from the body or take hours and hours to break down and convert into usable fuel. They aren't laden with fat, cholesterol, added sugars, or sodium. They are hydrating, nourishing, and nutrient-dense. When picking a food for a detox, ask yourself: Is this food nutrient-dense? How many ingredients does it have? (Hopefully just one.)

Anyone who's ever been addicted to drugs, cigarettes, or alcohol knows addiction in general is a very negative thing. Food happens to be one of the most potent "drugs" around. Unlike the case with other drugs, you need food to survive, which makes choosing the right food for your body and health extremely difficult in a world that thrusts unhealthy options in your face with every TV commercial, billboard, and fast-food restaurant chain. It can seem un-American to refrain from eating hamburgers, hot dogs, and pizzas. Everyone is doing it. Why shouldn't you?

Nutrition Density: More Bang for the Buck

Nutrient density refers to the ratio of nutrient content to the total energy content. Most often, foods without an ingredient list (fruits, veggies, legumes, nuts, seeds, grains, etc.) are nutrient-dense foods. Packaged foods that have a list of ten ingredients are usually lacking in nutrients and instead full of fillers like added oil, salt, sugar, chemicals, and preservatives. Our bodies are not made to digest these foods. They have been put together by machines and are designed to make us fat, tired, sick, and inevitably want more.

While we are able to digest a plethora of items and store the rest as fat, damage is done along the way. Heart disease is still the number one killer of women in this country. Why? Stress, inactivity, and poor food choices.

People often brag about how much they're eating and give you a hard time if you're not indulging as well. "I don't want to eat that rabbit food," I've often heard. But that "rabbit" food can taste great, slash disease, and give you an energetic, healthy life—which is just what the doctor ordered if you plan on having a baby.

Improved Digestion

Digestion is an exhaustive process, taking anywhere from 40 to 50 hours from start to finish! Think about what the body goes through to digest a single piece of fruit. Now throw in a heavy steak dinner, wine, and dessert at the end of a day in which you've already ingested food. Your body is constantly breaking food down instead of spending that energy healing and repairing. Where do you think all of your energy goes? To your gut.

When you think about your activity level versus what you ingest (especially on those enjoyable nights out dining with friends and family), you may grossly overestimate the amount of calories you burn in any given day. One hour of exercise can be "undone" with a muffin and a latte. And what if that food gets stuck in your gut, if your arteries become clogged, or your colon isn't doing its jobs at elimination? That translates into a lot of waste in the system—waste that needs to be removed for a fully functioning digestive tract.

If you love bread, cheese, butter, oil, sugar, and meat, these foods can slow down your digestion and make your colon useless for elimination. A healthy colon can eliminate two to four times per day! If you're not eliminating the food you're eating, you are storing it. Food, especially animal protein, can putrefy and rot in your digestive tract. You want to focus on food in and food out. This is why fiber-rich whole foods that flush toxins from our systems are so important.

Every time you digest something, there's a damage response. There's friction—squeezing, churning, and pushing. So, digestion is an event in and of itself. When you eat clean, fibrous food, you allow the body to more efficiently do its job, remove toxin buildup, and move things along, all while allowing your system to absorb vital nutrients and minerals from healthier, more easily digestible fare.

We have gotten away from thinking of our food as fuel. It's become a luxury, a crutch, an indulgence, or an enemy. Historically, we ate food to give us energy, to keep our systems functioning properly, and quite simply, to survive. With the current obesity pandemic, it's evident we are not eating for survival. We are living to eat.

It takes years of unhealthy food and lifestyle choices to result in disease. It also takes a bit of time to undo some of that damage, but we can start immediately if we are willing to make a few healthy dietary swaps.

Set Your Child Up with a Healthy Lifestyle

Studying children is a prime example of where our energy levels *should* be. Children generally have an abundance of energy; they have clear, healthy skin, bright eyes, and healthy joints, even when we feed them fast food, soda, and sugar-laden treats. It can take years until these dietary choices manifest into health issues, but they *will* manifest if not reversed.

According to statistics published in the *Journal of American Medical Association* and the Centers for Disease Control and Prevention, childhood obesity has more than doubled in children and quadrupled in adolescents in the past 30 years. Even more alarming? In 2012, more than one-third of children and adolescents were overweight or obese! Starting your child with healthy foods in the womb can set him or her up for a life of healthier options and a clean bill of health down the road. Instead of fast food, give them the option of healthy whole foods so they can adjust their taste buds to real food and not the modern conveniences of our fast-food lives.

Plants and Vegetables Deliver Nutrition

Most whole-foods detoxification programs focus on nutrient-dense foods, which are usually plants. Why? Because fruits and vegetables are easy to digest and are nutritionally dense, which means less nutritional stress and debt on the body. These whole foods heal the body and repair damage on a cellular level. What deters many people from eating more plant-based foods (and what hinders some vegans and vegetarians from reaching optimal levels of health) is that they focus on what they are avoiding rather than what to include in the diet. They focus so much on avoiding meat or dairy that they forget or neglect the abundance of food you can eat. Because overdosing on fresh foods is difficult, they can offer the body the break it requires. This way of eating puts the body into a state of detox, naturally.

But you might ask the inevitable question: What about protein? While a steak can give you plenty of iron and protein, it doesn't provide much else. You are also eating what that animal had eaten—usually a constant diet of corn or other nutritionally devoid food (parasites included). A fistful of organic kale on the other hand? You'll get protein (all greens have protein), vitamins, minerals, antioxidants, and fiber—all for a fraction of the cost of that filet. So yes, you can get enough protein while on a whole-foods, plant-based detoxification program.

The Protein Myth

We are a nation obsessed with protein. A meal is incomplete if it doesn't have protein as the center star. We are taught that to get strong, we have to have protein, and that protein must come from an animal. But times, they are a-changing.

People are starting to understand that our bodies do not, in fact, need copious amounts of protein to thrive. In fact, it's quite the opposite. We consume vastly too much protein, which wreaks havoc on our livers and causes our bodies to become more acidic (which is where disease thrives). Not only is animal protein acidic, it can be incredibly hard to digest.

Swap that meat-centered meal with a plant-based meal, and you can have it in and out of your system in a matter of hours. A piece of meat? It can take up to four days to digest! But what about "complete" proteins—those proteins that contain all of the essential amino acids? Most vegetables contain not only the essential amino acids, but all of the amino acids.

Does this mean you have to be vegan on this program? Absolutely not. But, if you choose to eat meat while detoxing, pay attention to where your meat comes from and opt for organic, local protein sources whenever possible. Check your local farmers' markets or CSAs (community supported agriculture) and talk to vendors and farmers about their animal practices.

The benefits of plant-based proteins are endless. They are cheaper and easier to digest and most can be eaten raw, so you can save time in the kitchen. They are ideal when detoxifying the body, giving the liver a break and helping to cleanse the system. If you have years of buildup, it makes sense to give the body a break, right? If you are someone who thinks you can't live without meat, this is an opportunity to see how you feel eating the right foods while cutting out animal protein. Even a span of ten days to two weeks will reap health benefits, allowing the digestive system to expel toxins and heal. However, I recommend a period of six weeks for a plant-based diet to do its job.

You can still be fit and strong and eat less protein (yes, really) and focus on all of the other nutrients and minerals you need, especially when it comes to preparing your body for pregnancy. The general recommendation for protein?

Your weight x .35 +10 (once pregnant) = X grams

For example, if I weigh 135 pounds, I would multiply 135 x .35 = 45.5 grams of protein per day. Once pregnant, I would add 10 grams, which equals 55.5 grams of protein per day. With these calculations, you can see how easy it is to get enough protein spread throughout the day.

Take a Bite: We Are Designed to Eat Plants

It's important to look at human physiology in relation to the types of foods we are meant to eat versus what we have come, in this society, to deem as normal.

Unless you fantasize about eating birds or ripping a cow apart with your bare hands, you are probably more of an omnivore or herbivore than a strict carnivore. From our very small, blunt canine teeth to our hands with their soft fingernails, we aren't meant to kill large prey.

While carnivores have jaws that move only up and down, humans are able to move their jaws from side to side as well, which allows us to grind food with our back teeth. Many scientists suggest our teeth are made specifically for grinding fibrous plant foods.

According to anthropologist Dr. Richard Leakey in *The Natural Human Diet*, our anterior teeth are not suited for tearing flesh or hide. We don't have large canine teeth, and we wouldn't have been able to deal with food sources that require those large canines.

While most carnivores can swallow their food whole due to their stomach acids' ability to break down food and kill bacteria, our systems are not as acidic. Our longer intestines allow the body to break down fiber and absorb nutrients. When we eat a lot of meat, bacteria can get caught in our digestive tracts and make us sick.

Carnivores of the animal kingdom don't suffer from heart disease or cancer or get sore after running to kill prey. In eating food our bodies weren't meant to digest (and this goes well beyond meat), humans pay the consequences. Dr. Leakey says:

> Human bodies were not designed to process animal flesh, so all the excess fat and cholesterol from a meat-based diet makes us sick. Heart disease is the number one killer in America according to the American Heart Association, and medical experts agree that this ailment is largely the result of the consumption of animal products. Meat-eaters have a 50 percent higher risk of developing heart disease than vegetarians!

So, why do we consume so much protein? Advertising, baby. It's what we are made to believe we have to eat: milk (for calcium) and meat (for protein). We laugh if our toddlers won't eat their veggies and give them chicken nuggets instead. We let them eat cake and ice cream and drink Cokes with their fast-food hamburgers. We shrug and say, "It's just what kids eat!" Is it? Should it be?

Animal protein raises the acidity level in the blood, causing calcium to be excreted from the bones to restore the blood's natural pH balance. This calcium depletion leads to osteoporosis, and the excreted calcium ends up in the kidneys, where it can form kidney stones or even trigger kidney disease.

Historically, only the wealthy ate animals. Ironically, rich people who ingested animal protein were the ones most likely to be plagued with disease. So, the bottom line is this: Don't eat out of habit. Eat from knowledge. While it might not be feasible for you to give up meat, eat it in moderation. You definitely don't need it with every meal (and neither does your baby). Focus your meal around veggies and other whole foods instead.

Use the steps in this book to make more educated choices and enjoy a few plant-based days to see how much better you feel!

The Importance of Alkaline Foods

If you partake in a semi-traditional American diet, chances are your system might be acidic. Attempting to bring more alkaline foods into the body is imperative to restoring the balance. When you think of alkalinity, think of donating minerals to the body. Alkaline foods donate minerals, while acidic foods steal minerals. Unfortunately, so many of the foods we love are acidic: caffeine, sugar, meat, dairy, wheat, etc.

Upping your plant-based foods and reducing acidic foods not only restores your alkaline balance but also provides you with an abundance of energy.

Which foods have the highest alkalinity point? The options are many. Choose from most leafy greens, broccoli, cabbage, carrots, celery, chlorella, garlic, onions, fermented veggies, peppers, tomatoes, sweet potatoes, sea veggies, mushrooms, apples, avocados, bananas, most berries, coconut, dates, grapefruit, lemons, limes, almonds, fermented soy, cinnamon, ginger, all herbs, apple cider vinegar, blackstrap molasses, and probiotic cultures, to start.

Many healthy foods we love, such as blueberries, plums, amaranth, barley, bread, oatmeal, quinoa, spelt, almond milk, black beans, garbanzo beans, lentils, soy milk, butter, cheese, ice cream, cashews, peanut butter, pecans, tahini, and most animal proteins register as acidic.

This doesn't mean you should avoid these foods entirely. It's important to maintain a balance. You can't *only* eat alkaline foods. The pH scale ranges from 0 to 14. Seven is in the middle, which makes it neutral (neither acid or alkaline). The lower the number, the more acidic a substance. For instance, hydrochloric acid has a pH of 0, as it's the most acidic a substance can get. Distilled water would be neutral at 7. The higher the number, the more alkaline; however, you do not want to be on the high or low end of the pH scale. For example, bleach has a pH of 13 (extremely alkaline). We want to stay in that slightly alkaline range (7.35–7.45).

You can study foods to see where they fall on the pH scale. However, understand that certain foods like apple cider vinegar and lemon juice, which are acidic, actually have a very alkaline effect in the body. It's important to know where you are on the pH scale and how the food you're eating affects your body. To see a full list of alkaline and acidic foods, pick up my book *Power Vegan*.

If you're interested in finding out your pH, grab a test at your local health food store and see where you register on the pH scale!

Remember that it's not just food that contributes to an acidic environment. Stress, emotional exhaustion, drugs, and alcohol all contribute. This detox is about food, yes, but also bringing the stress down in other areas of your life, eliminating unhealthy behaviors, and readying your mind and body to conceive.

Navigating Pesticides

Does it really matter if you choose organic or conventionally grown fruits and veggies?

As discussed in the juicing section on page 21, purchasing local and organic as much as possible is vital to ridding the body of potential toxins, especially in the way of insecticides and pesticides. There are many schools of thought on pesticides, because when the crop is sprayed and how much is used is always up for debate, not to mention how little is left on the fruit or vegetable by the time it's ready to be sold. This is why it's important to talk to farmers who do use pesticides to find out just how much they use and when they use it (especially if you can't afford organic). It is good to note, however, that damaged organic produce—meaning fruits or veggies that have perforated skin or seem damaged—actually have a higher toxicity than pesticide-sprayed produce due to the length of the natural defense of a chemical's half-life, or the amount of time it takes for a chemical compound potency to break down. Man-made pesticides are chemically engineered to dissipate, but organic compounds are hardier. Johnny Cooke explains:

> Anything living has a defense response. When you damage the skin, it has its own defense system. Plants will produce their own pesticide to kill off invaders. They have an immune system almost mimicking ours. The toxins they produce to kill off invaders can and will be ingested if we eat damaged organic produce, which can have less-than-favorable effects.

Bottom line? Make sure you purchase unblemished organic produce and consume it within a few days to ensure the best quality of nutrients. Dr. Steven Pratt, author of *SuperFoods Rx for Pregnancy,* explains:

> Insecticides are essentially neurotoxins. Once they enter the food supply, and the mothers' bodies, it seems likely that their neurotoxicity may be a risk to a developing human nervous system. Studies of cord blood in newborns have shown over 200 xenobiotics and chemicals, and new-to-nature molecules that bathe the emerging infant. Our environment has changed radically. Foods are now highly processed, pesticides and insecticides in them are common, chemicals from plastics disrupt vital hormonal pathways, and nutrient deficiencies alter expression of genes and increase birth defects.

So how do you know which foods to reach for and which to avoid? The Environmental Working Group put together the latest list of the top forty-eight foods that were dirtiest to cleanest, as well as an updated version of the "dirty dozen" and the "clean fifteen." The dirty dozen, which are conventional fruits and veggies, were found to contain at least forty-seven different chemicals. When you ingest these chemicals, they wreak havoc on the body (and if pregnant, possibly the fetus). When purchasing the produce on the dirty dozen list, always opt for organic; avoid them altogether if organic isn't an option.

2014 Dirty Dozen

1. Apples
2. Strawberries
3. Grapes
4. Celery
5. Peaches
6. Spinach
7. Sweet bell peppers
8. Nectarines (imported)
9. Cucumbers
10. Cherry tomatoes
11. Snap peas (imported)
12. Potatoes

If you can't afford organic produce, the "clean fifteen" contain lower to no traces of pesticides and are considered safe to consume in conventional form.

2014 Clean Fifteen

1. Avocados
2. Sweet corn
3. Pineapples
4. Cabbage
5. Sweet peas (frozen)
6. Onions
7. Asparagus
8. Mangos
9. Papayas
10. Kiwis
11. Eggplant
12. Grapefruit
13. Cantaloupe
14. Cauliflower
15. Sweet potatoes

It's good to note that both of these lists were compiled after the USDA had high-pressure washed both sets of produce. It is vital to wash produce (whether conventional or organic), even if the produce has a thick skin, like some of the produce listed on the clean list.

While detoxing through food is imperative, detoxing your lifestyle and environment before you conceive can help increase your chances of a healthy pregnancy, delivery, and beyond. *Detox Before You're Expecting* aims to help you address all areas of your life while cutting out some of the junk.

Just take it one balanced step at a time.

CHAPTER THREE

Why Detox Before Pregnancy?

Babies do not enter this world with a clean slate. The state of your health at the time of conception becomes your child's "go" point. The weaker your cells and organs, the more your baby will suffer. Because of our country's current state of health, genetics, and the influences of toxic environments, kids are developing "adult" diseases like cancer and diabetes. Everything you eat, breathe, and do has a positive or negative effect on your body (and when you become pregnant, your baby). When you start to look at every choice you make in these terms, food just doesn't look the same. A cookie is no longer a cookie. A beer is no longer just a beer.

Of course, there's always a laissez-faire approach—this usually introduces a slew of avoidable pregnancy symptoms, unhealthy weight gain, and complicated deliveries. But pregnancy does *not* have to be impossible or gross or miserable. You do not have to gain fifty pounds and crave ice cream for dinner.

There is another way.

You wouldn't get up today and decide, "Hey! I'm going to run a marathon this afternoon!" So, why would you think you could just hop into pregnancy unprepared? A marathon, by comparison, is easy compared to what the body goes through when pregnant. From stretching ligaments and joints to organs moving out of the way to make room for a growing baby, increased bloodflow, and changes in your body odor, skin, hair, hormones, and appetite, this is one of the most taxing events your body will endure.

With symptoms like acid reflux, intense nausea, skin rashes, and stretch marks, it can be a challenging time to care about what you put in your mouth when there are so many other factors to worry about. So you indulge. Suddenly, a few "cheats" here and there start to add up until you have gained fifty pounds and you think, "Oh well! I'm pregnant. If there was ever a time to indulge, it's now."

Gaining a bit of self-control before you're pregnant can help shift your mindset when curbing those pregnancy cravings or when your hormones make you want to eat a house.

Balancing Hormonal Fluctuations

Hormonal fluctuation happens all the time and for numerous reasons. With interference from the likes of birth control to chemicals to the foods we eat, once this "life force" gets out of whack, conception can be greatly hindered. Assessing your hormones from your doctor or a holistic practitioner can give you a good starting point for the work you need to do. The good news? Oftentimes, cleansing the body can do this for you—naturally.

Besides wanting yourself and your baby to be healthy, there are many reasons to cleanse your body before pregnancy. As

Nina Nelson explains in her online article "How and Why You Should Cleanse or Detoxify Before Pregnancy," cleansing and detoxifying the body are most often used to balance body pH, lose weight, jump-start healing, stop cravings, increase energy, relieve allergies, increase chances of conception, and balance hormones.

Feeding the Fetus

Baby Centre UK explains how the food you eat reaches the baby:

> Once the food travels down mom's esophagus, it moves to her stomach, where it will be broken down into fats, glucose, and protein. After digestion, the food will be absorbed into the blood and passed from mother to child through the placenta. This is a very efficient filter that weeds out harmful bacteria that can harm the fetus. Smaller elements can pass through the barrier, however—oxygen, glucose, fats, protein, vitamins, minerals, as well as caffeine and alcohol. After these elements have entered the bloodstream, they pass to the fetus through the umbilical cord.

One of the simplest ways to avoid passing chemicals or toxins to a fetus? Change your diet. Eating a healthy diet is critical to fetal development and a mother's health during pregnancy. When you stop to think about it, it makes perfect sense. Healthy mama equals healthy baby. Even if you don't eat great, what better time to start? For the first time in your life, eating is serving a dual purpose—it's about nourishment *and* enjoyment (which is hard to remember when you're ravenous or throwing up).

The Academy of Nutrition and Dietetics recommends that pregnant women consume 2,200 to 2,900 calories daily, increasing intake gradually as pregnancy progresses. This amount, of course, varies if you are overweight or underweight. Generally, you will eat extra calories with each trimester. Below are suggestions for extra calories per day.

FIRST TRIMESTER	0 extra calories (unless you are underweight)
SECOND TRIMESTER	250–350 extra calories
THIRD TRIMESTER	350–450 extra calories

While overeating can be a problem during pregnancy, poor nutrition can be a major factor in improper fetal development as well. Research published in the *Journal of Nutrition* found that poor maternal nutrition changes gene expression in fetuses of laboratory animals, suggesting that a mother's poor diet may alter how fetal genes function.

Bottom line? It's vital to get healthy before you conceive to give you and your baby the easiest pregnancy and delivery possible.

Preventing Pregnancy Complications

In addition to a balanced diet, is there a way to prevent pregnancy complications? According to the National Institute of Child Health and Human Development, there are numerous risk factors for pre-term labor and birth, which include (but are not limited to):

- Abnormalities of the reproductive organs
- Urinary tract infections
- Sexually transmitted infections (STIs)
- High blood pressure
- Being underweight or obese
- Diabetes
- Age of the mother (younger than eighteen or older than thirty-five)

- No health care (or late health care during pregnancy)
- Smoking
- Drinking alcohol
- Using drugs
- Abuse
- Lack of social support
- Stress
- Exposure to environmental pollutants

Addressing any avoidable issues prior to pregnancy is important in helping you enjoy these forty weeks.

While many of us can have problem areas we need to detox, generally the colon, lymph, liver, and kidneys take the brunt of the abuse we put our bodies through. The liver is the detox "mecca" of your body and attempts to filter and remove the toxins (as do the kidneys). The lymph keeps all those toxins moving through the body, unless they become congested. It's important when detoxifying to address these organs and get them as clean as possible prior to pregnancy, since your body will be asked to work overtime if any of these organs or systems are compromised.

The Liver

The entire purpose of the liver is to remove toxins from the blood. It also processes proteins, nutrients, cholesterol, and glucose. Constantly eating poor foods and drinking alcohol damages the liver (though this is the only organ that *can* regenerate). Many people swear by dandelion, milk thistle, and turmeric (perfect for a tea) to help cleanse the liver. Other great foods to eat for liver detoxification are:

- Artichokes
- Asparagus
- Avocados
- Basil
- Beets
- Broccoli
- Brussels sprouts
- Cabbage
- Carrots
- Garlic
- Grapefruits
- Onions

- Sesame seeds
- Spinach (Those who are sensitive to oxalic acid should avoid spinach or other greens that contain oxalates. They can cause kidney and gallbladder stones.)
- Tomatoes
- Walnuts

The Kidneys

The kidneys filter out toxins, as well as excess salt. They also filter blood, produce urine, and regulate acid (which is why it's so important to not eat an overabundance of acidic foods).

One of the easiest ways to keep the kidneys healthy is to cut back on excess salt and to start your day with a hot cup of water with lemon. Lemon helps rid the body of toxins and helps flush them from the system prior to breakfast.

The following healthy-kidney foods are suggested by Pauline Hanuise in *How to Support and Detox Your Kidneys*:

- Asparagus
- Baking soda
- Barley
- Black currant juice
- Blueberries
- Cranberry juice
- Dandelion tea
- Ginger
- Grapes
- Lemon juice
- Marshmallow root
- Millet
- Nettle tea
- Parsley
- Pumpkin seeds
- Red clover
- Spirulina
- Turmeric
- Watermelon

The Lymphatic System

Think of your lymphatic system as your transportation center. The lymphatic system collects fats, tissue fluids, and even enzymes and hormones and gets them where they need to go.

This system also filters out bacteria and other toxins, which is why it's vital to keep it healthy. It is imperative to exercise for a healthy lymphatic system, as well as to drink enough water. Lymphatic massage can help with getting things "moving" along, as can staying away from processed foods that encourage blockages. Often when the lymph is sluggish, the skin is dull, agitated, or broken out. When you feed your lymphatic system with healthy foods, the skin almost always improves. Here are some foods that promote a healthy lymphatic system:

- Apples
- Apricots
- Bananas
- Cranberries
- Dates
- Dark green vegetables
- Dried figs
- Flaxseeds

- Garlic
- Ginger
- Kelp
- Lemons
- Oranges
- Raisins
- Radishes
- Wheatgrass

The Colon

Chances are you've probably had colon issues at one time or another in your life. The colon (or large intestine) removes water, salt, and some nutrients from food and forms stool. Billions of bacteria coat the colon, which is why it's vital that when we flush these bacteria out, we put them back in balance with probiotics. Many people suffer from colon issues, from intermittent diarrhea to Crohn's disease, colitis, polyps, etc. So much of our colon issues can be fixed by cutting out the inflammatory foods in our diets (meat, dairy, and processed foods) and consuming easier-to-digest foods in their natural state. Healing your colon before pregnancy should be on the top of your list, especially if you suffer from any issues. Try these foods:

- Apple cider vinegar
- Avocados
- Blueberries
- Brown rice
- Chia seeds
- Fennel
- Garlic
- Grapes
- Ginger
- Greens
- Fermented foods (these are full of probiotics to help heal the gut)
- Flaxseeds (ground)
- Pineapple
- Salmon
- Water with sea salt (Often, we don't drink enough to flush the toxins from our system. Making sure you are adequately hydrated helps protect the colon and allows it to better do its job.)
- White tea

As you'll find, many of these foods cross over. Whole foods are diverse in their ability to heal and detoxify the system. This is the type of nutrition our bodies crave, and in order to detox, we must step away from the typical American fare and give our bodies the chance to do what they do best: detox.

The Skinny

Take a look at your diet as it stands now, as well as some of the "bad" habits you may have that might hinder conception. Do you smoke? Do you drink more than two alcoholic beverages a week? Do you suck down caffeine like it's your best friend? Do you crave sugar every day of your life? Remember: This is not a quick fix. Knowing your habits and coming up with a detailed plan on how to alter or kick them for good is paramount to fulfilling a cleansing program and making lasting lifestyle changes.

Only you can commit to changing your life and your body. Getting a grasp on your health before you bring someone else into this world is one of the greatest gifts you can give your child.

CHAPTER FOUR

Why Your Partner Should Detox Too

My husband and I still marvel that our daughter came from his *balls*. How could two hanging glands and one egg create the most amazing human we could ever imagine? I am convinced that my husband's nutrition and fitness helped with what I call an "instant" conception. I am also convinced that my husband's antioxidant-rich diet coupled with slashing environmental pollutants contributed to an easy conception and healthy baby. It wasn't just about *my* health—it was about his too.

So it's time, ladies. For once, you can blame the health of your child and your ability to get pregnant on the man! Yes, you are the vessel for this life-changing journal, but a man's sperm can dictate the health of the child just as much as a woman's egg.

The American Pregnancy Association finds that male fertility factors contribute to approximately 50 percent of all infertility cases, and male infertility alone accounts for approximately one-third of all infertility cases. Steven Pratt writes in *SuperFoods Rx for Pregnancy*:

> Several studies suggest that semen quality is declining worldwide as a result of the increased exposure to endocrine disruptors, which are environmental chemicals that interfere with the synthesis, secretion, transport, binding, action, or elimination of natural hormones in the body. These disruptors may be found in water, soil, air, food, plastic containers, household products, and personal care products. Among the most widely implicated offenders are organochlorines, polychlorinated biphenyls (PCBs), dioxins, phthalates, pesticides, and herbicides.

Many factors go into getting pregnant. Start simply. Have your partner look at his diet and see where it could improve. The sperm he produces today was "made" 90 days ago, so paying attention now will ensure healthy sperm down the line. The following lifestyle changes can up your odds of conception:

- **MAKE AN APPOINTMENT WITH YOUR DOC.** This will rule out any serious conditions, genetic issues, or underlying problems.

- **AIM FOR A HEALTHY WEIGHT.** Just as with women, being underweight or overweight can have an adverse effect on a man's fertility and a growing fetus.

- **BOOST ZINC INTAKE.** Studies have shown that some men with low sperm count also have a zinc deficiency. To help remedy this, opt for amaranth, beans, bran flakes, brown rice, buckwheat, nutritional yeast, nuts, peas, pumpkin seeds, quinoa, spinach, tempeh or tofu, wheat germ, wild rice, seafood, and eggs.

- **BOOST VITAMIN E AND SELENIUM (FOUND IN BRAZIL NUTS) INTAKE.** This can also increase fertility odds.

- **FOLIC ACID ISN'T JUST FOR LADIES.** Men who had lower levels of folic acid in their diets had a higher rate of abnormal chromosomes in their sperm, according to Parents.com. When sperm with abnormal chromosomes fertilize an egg, it may result in miscarriage or birth defects. More than half of first-trimester miscarriages are caused by chromosomal abnormalities in the embryo. While men can take a multivitamin or even a prenatal (yes, really!), opting for foods high in folate, such as dark, leafy greens, legumes, nutritional yeast, orange juice, pseudograins, citrus fruits, and whole grains will help maintain a healthy amount of folic acid.

- **ELIMINATE CIGARETTES, ALCOHOL, CAFFEINE, SODA, MARI-JUANA, AND ANY OTHER DRUGS OR PILLS.** This is imperative prior to conception. Alcohol and drugs can decrease sperm quality and have a negative effect on a fetus. Big beer drinker? Come up with a plan to taper off alcohol before trying to conceive. According to Suzanne Kavic, MD, director of the division of reproductive endocrinology at Loyola University Health System, "Sperm production takes about three months, so any changes the man makes today won't show up in the semen for at least three months."

- **RECONSIDER YOUR MEDICATIONS.** One of the most overlooked issues with fertility? The use of certain medications and their interference with trying to conceive. Which medications have been known to impact fertility? The American Pregnancy Association indicates Tagamet (cimetidine), sulfasalazine, nitrofurantoin, steroids, such as prednisone and cortisone, and chemotherapy and radiation can cause sterility or a significant change in sperm quality and quantity. All of these medications may impact sperm production and sperm count.

- **IF YOUR MAN WORKS WITH CHEMICALS, IT MIGHT BE A GOOD TIME TO TAKE A BREAK OR USE THE PROPER PRECAUTIONARY METHODS, SUCH AS A MASK.** According to the National Institute of Occupational Safety and Health, ongoing exposure to pesticides, chemical fertilizers, lead, nickel, mercury, chromium, ethylene glycol ethers, petrochemicals, benzene, perchloroethylene, and radiation can lower sperm quality and quantity and possibly lead to infertility or miscarriage.

- **EXTREME HEAT (SUCH AS SAUNAS, HOT TUBS, AND EVEN LAPTOPS) CAN CAUSE THE TESTICLES TO OVERHEAT AND DECREASE SPERM.** This goes for sports such as cycling or marathon running, or any others that might cause injury or intense heat to that part of the body.

- **CUT OUT STRESS.** Stress, while not something you can easily "cut out" of your life, has a huge impact on overall well-being and the ability to conceive. Reducing stress, improving sleep quality, a healthy diet, and getting plenty of exercise can prime your partner's body (and yours) for conception. Diet and lifestyle changes at least three months prior to conception is optimal.

The Skinny

Think of this journey as something you and your partner can do together. If you want to start a family, use it as an excuse to "spring clean" your diets, lifestyle choices, and environmental toxins. Look at it as a joint effort, and commit yourselves to helping each other through this incredibly exciting time in both your lives.

CHAPTER FIVE

What Kind of Detox Do You Need?

One of the sneakiest culprits in our daily lives is processed food. "But I don't eat a lot of processed food," you might say. You might want to think again. Go look at your pantry and fridge right now. If you have pasta, cereals, or crackers on your shelves, you eat processed food. If you open your fridge and find anything in a package or container, you eat processed foods. From the condiments you eat to the bread you slather them on, these foods have gone through a process to make them "edible," which sometimes means being pumped full of everything under the kitchen sink. Even if you're a "healthy" eater, you probably eat more processed foods than you think (myself included). If you buy nondairy milk, tofu, protein bars, coffee, granola, hummus, yogurt, or bread, you are eating processed foods. Now, how often do you ingest these foods?

Every day? When you have a salad, do you throw anything on top of it that's come from a package?

If most of your meals revolve around processed foods, you have a bit more detoxing to do. One of the easiest ways to prep yourself for a cleanse is to replace one processed food with one fresh food (which is easier than you think). Yes, some "shifting" of the taste buds will be involved, but most of what we eat is either out of convenience or habit. Chances are you can handle a collard green as a burrito wrap, or making your own almond milk instead of purchasing it at the store. Stay aware of areas you can swap in fresh foods for processed.

While we are creatures of habit, often our bodies give signals when they need a detox. Symptoms can be wide and varying, but can correlate to different parts of your body. You can use some sort of detoxification if you experience any of these symptoms, as noted by Jeffrey Morrison in *Cleanse Your Body, Clear Your Mind*:

Common Symptoms

- Painful menstrual cycles or fertility issues
- Genital itch or discharge
- Hot flashes
- Night sweats
- Loss of libido
- Lethargy
- Fatigue
- Restlessness
- Insomnia
- Anxiety
- Depression
- Mood swings
- Headache
- Under-eye circles
- Watery or itchy eyes
- Earaches
- Itchy ears
- Excessive nasal mucus
- Hay fever
- Sinus problems
- Sneezing
- Stuffy nose
- Canker sores
- Coughing
- Sore throat
- Acne
- Flushing

- Hives
- Rashes
- Dry skin
- Asthma
- Bronchitis
- Chest congestion
- Joint aches
- Stiffness
- Belching

- Passing gas
- Bloating
- Constipation
- Diarrhea
- Heartburn
- Intestinal/stomach pain
- Nausea
- Frequent illness

Less Common Symptoms

- Confusion
- Difficulty making decisions
- Poor memory
- Slurred speech
- Stuttering
- Dizziness
- Faintness
- Tunnel vision
- Swollen eyelids
- Drainage from ears
- Gagging
- Hoarseness
- Swollen tongue, gums, or lips

- Excessive sweating
- Hair loss
- Difficulty breathing
- Shortness of breath
- Arthritis
- Weakness
- Vomiting
- Chest pain
- Frequent urination
- Irregular heartbeat
- Rapid or pounding heart
- Numbness or tingling in hands or feet

This is an exhaustive list. (Some of these symptoms are more severe than others and should require medical attention to rule out other illnesses.) Despite popular belief, we are not supposed to suffer from so many of the common ailments we associate with being human. From allergies to stomach issues to bad body odor, many common disturbances can be eradicated by cleansing the system safely and effectively. Some of the most widely felt symptoms people experience on a daily basis are unexplained fatigue, sluggish elimination, irritated skin, allergies, low-grade infections, puffy eyes or bags under the eyes, menstrual problems, and mental fog (fuzzy-headedness). Taking inventory of your own issues, name your top ten biggest complaints. As you venture into this detox, see which ones linger and which ones disappear (and which ones might not be correlated to food). Ever been stressed? This can wreak havoc on every part of your body. Drowning yourself in chemicals with the lotions you use and the makeup you wear? You could be toxifying yourself from the outside in. It's all connected.

Determining Your Detox Plan

If you know your physical issues, how do you know what kind of detox you really need? First, ask yourself the following questions.

1. On a scale of one to ten, how healthy am I now?

2. How often do I get sick and visit the doctor?

3. Do I suffer from menstrual issues or gastrointestinal problems?

4. Would I describe myself as healthy?

5. How physically active am I?

6. How regularly do I eliminate?

7. Do I suffer from skin problems via breakouts or rashes (on face, back, shoulders, etc.)?

8. Do I ever get bouts of diarrhea, constipation, gas, or bloating from something I ate?

9. Do I wake up tired on most days?

10. Do I have dark circles under my eyes?

Study your answers. Where could improvements be made? Where have you tried to make improvements before and failed?

What hinders you with leading the healthy life you want? Knowing where your hang-ups are can drastically increase your odds of lasting success if you are honest with yourself and any shortcomings. Getting healthy is a gradual process.

Pre-pregnancy and pregnancy are generally not times to start a new exercise regimen or diet. A safe whole-foods detoxification program is *not* a diet. You will be cleansing the body in preparation for pregnancy. There's a distinction between preparing your body and dieting.

The following detoxes are divided into three areas: beginner, intermediate, and advanced. The more issues you have and the less healthy your diet and lifestyle are, the more you should stick to the beginner detox. You want to start slowly and give your body a chance to adjust as best as possible. Read on to find which area you fit in best.

Beginner: There's Still Hope!

You love a standard American diet. Commercials with cheeseburgers and pizza make your eyes glaze and your mouth water. You have been known to hit the fast food drive-through in the middle of the night if the craving strikes. You eat what you want, when you want. Your idea of a healthy meal might be skipping the butter, but that's about it.

You want to get healthy, but you don't want to give up all the foods you love. You may have tried diets, but the moment your favorite foods are banned, you hoard them and stuff your face just to prove a point: You can do what you want.

To you, most health foods taste like cardboard, and you don't have the time or money to buy organic or try disgusting kale chips or eat anything green. You love your milkshakes and desserts and fried chicken, and you'll be damned if taking all of that away is going to be easy.

You take or have taken medications. You have suffered from skin issues, gastrointestinal issues, common colds and flus, etc. For you, it's just part of life. You haven't really known another way.

But, you know that health is important, especially if you want to have a baby. Maybe you are overweight or even appear to be a healthy weight, but you may be suffering from several ailments—many of which could be eliminated with dietary changes. So, because of that, you *are* willing to try...maybe.

The first step for you is to eliminate what's been built up in your system for so long. Sometimes, this requires a bit more than eating healthy food. By eating more of the right foods, your system will be able to clean out what's been stored and accumulated. However, once you begin eating healthier, if you feel you are up for it, researching enemas or colonics would be beneficial to "empty the tank," so to speak.

For you, transitioning into healthier foods the *right* way is vital; otherwise, it will feel like deprivation and you won't last. Your process will take longer, and because of this, a two-week omission period is recommended to prepare your body for detoxification, a two-week transition period, and then a four-week clean eating period. Eight weeks of your life to help prep for baby. Not bad.

Intermediate: I'm on the Right Track!

You know what healthy food is. You eat well around 50 percent of the time, but if you want a decadent meal, you're going to have it, and guilt will not follow. You've been known to try diets or the newest craze, but eventually, you stop and revert back to your comfort zone. You're about moderation, even if that moderation means binge eating for three days and then getting back on track for the rest of the week. You tend to buy the same things in the grocery store, because you like them and you know they taste good.

You're open-minded and genuinely like the taste of healthy food. You just don't want to be boxed into one label.

You can eat a quinoa dish or steak and potatoes. You don't discriminate and enjoy most food. You would consider yourself healthy, but you know your diet and your body could use a bit of improvement, and you are willing and able to ensure a healthy pregnancy and delivery. You get the occasional cold; you have your "issues" around that time of the month, and your skin and hair drive you crazy sometimes.

For you, a ten-day omission period to remove all trigger foods is recommended, followed by three weeks of "clean" eating. This thirty-one day process should be enough time to cleanse the organs and body and ready yourself for pregnancy.

Advanced: I'm Practically Perfect!

You almost didn't even buy this book. You make your own nondairy milk, you sprout your seeds and grains, and you bottle your own kombucha. You might even have a garden or frequent the farmers' market where people know you by name. In fact, you could probably *write* a book if you really wanted to. You're that in tune with your health. Though you eat healthy now, you might not have always eaten this way. Perhaps you indulged in processed, greasy fare and candy all throughout childhood. Perhaps you live in a very polluted environment or are under stress. You understand that being healthy is about more than what goes into your mouth. Though you're a great eater, you need more of a maintenance detox to make sure you're getting enough nutrients and are at a healthy weight before conception.

You want a healthy baby, and you're willing to do whatever it takes to get there.

A quick seven-day omission period (and "check in" to see what nutrients you may be lacking or what variety you can include into your daily diet) is recommended, followed by a two-week cleansing period. Twenty-one days should be all you need to ensure you're ready for baby.

Once you decide what category you are in, simply follow the step-by-step guide in Chapter Ten to help you detox and get ready for conception.

CHAPTER SIX

Changing the Way You Think About Food

Why do we eat? You might think of numerous responses. It's a time to be social. It's a time for comfort. It's a time to fuel your body for an activity, or to recover from one. But, at the end of the day, we eat for energy. Nothing else. We need food to stay alive, and *everything* we eat is broken down into usable energy.

However, what some of us eat the most (i.e., processed foods and a standard American diet) doesn't give us the right kind of energy. This is not only because of the types of foods we eat, but more importantly, the *amount*. For instance, if I were an ultra-marathon runner, I could probably down a large pizza and donuts while running 100 miles, and my body would use that energy. I would probably still be in a caloric deficit because of the amount of energy expended. I wouldn't suffer at the hands of the ingredients because none of that food—no matter how calorie dense—would be stored as fat and wreak havoc on my body. But I am not an ultra-marathon runner. Most of us are not elite endurance athletes, but some of us eat like we are.

While I'm not an endurance athlete, I've been an athlete all of my life, flitting from sport to sport. I would settle on gymnastics for thirteen years and competitive boxing for five. I've spent six days per week in the gym (even while pregnant) for the majority of my life. But, I am someone who has also grossly overconsumed calories to her heart's content. I used to make a sport out of eating, until I was past the point of comfort. I would clean my plate, going back for just one more helping and one more. I was a victim of food comas on all major holidays, clutching my stomach and declaring "I am never eating again."

I've always been able to relate to my clients who are "addicted" to food, because my mindset has always been hyperfocused on eating. My parents used to joke that I would not survive one day on a desert island, and they would be right. If I go too long without food, I become grumpy, tired, and overly dramatic, throwing out such words as "starving" and "going to die."

When I go to sleep, I think about breakfast. While I'm eating breakfast, I think about lunch. Nothing makes me happier than a full refrigerator, and the times in my life when I have been unsure how I was even going to pay my bills, I would not give up purchasing good, healthy food. To me, "enough" food has always represented a good quality of life. And then one day, it dawned on me: I want to collect memories, not Whole Foods Market receipts.

Now, I know better. I have come to realize that just because my head is screaming for me to eat that brownie (Just eat it! Just eat it! Just eat it!), I don't actually *need* it. I can sit and think about the way that I will feel, or how three giant bowls of brown rice pasta—however tasty—is simply going to be stored in my body as fat, since I'm going to do nothing but sit on the couch for the evening; but the mind, as we all know, is an incredibly powerful thing. So, how do we break the cycle?

Eating is a behavior, and behaviors are controlled and coordinated by the brain. We have to look at what behaviors we have when it comes to eating. Do you have patterns with eating? Do you continuously skip breakfast? Are you a late-night binge eater? Do you eat "well," but then all bets are off when you're out with your friends?

You have to know what your behaviors are now and what they've always been to have any chance of changing them. For me, I am open and willing to shift my views, my way of thinking and eating. But I always revert back to eating in a style that's comfortable for me. Now, that doesn't mean stuffing myself. But, it means eating well most of the time, and when I want to make cookies or I want to eat out, I will. Maybe I will exercise harder, reduce portions, or just get on with my day.

Daily needs and wants change, and I am "budgeting" for those changes. I am being realistic about what I can and can't do. Being realistic is the first key to your success.

Unlearning Traditions

What if everything surrounding food—from eating a nutritious breakfast to getting enough vitamin D to needing so many milligrams of calcium per day to making sure you're getting the right sources of protein—was all *learned*?

From the hunger pangs you think you feel (conditioned response!) to eating breakfast, lunch, and dinner at the same times each day to pairing certain foods together, you've learned the behavior from somewhere. It could be from your parents, television, friends, advertising, a favorite celebrity, the doctor, or leading experts. You are taking information someone else has given you and applying it to yourself because you *think* that this is the way to get healthy. It's what the diet and health industry wants. Try X and lose this much weight! Erase diabetes with the easiest diet you will ever try! Turn back time with these ten superfoods! But you have to learn to think for yourself.

As I've said to all of my clients at one time or another, we aren't born liking cake, cookies, and pizza. We learn to enjoy these foods from what we are exposed to. When we go to a birthday party, we know there will be cake. At the movies, we'll bury our hands in a bucket of buttery popcorn. On a hot summer night, we'll take the kids to get ice cream. What does any of this have to do with hunger? Nothing. It has much more to do with traditions. As people, we make traditions surrounding our food. Had a bad day? Let's eat chocolate. Endured a stressful week at work? Let's have a couple of beers. Excited for Super Bowl Sunday? Let's eat as much meat and chili as we can possibly consume! Taking your kid to a restaurant? Let's order mac and cheese and chicken fingers. And this is where the hard part comes in, because so much of the food we eat is surrounded by joy, family, memories, and most importantly, society's standards. Look at any other culture, and people around the world are brought together by food. It's one thing that unites us.

But that doesn't mean you should accept traditions just because they are passed down to you. I can't tell you how many times I've had to pepper the waiter with questions or ask for a simpler meal; or how many times I've been on a road trip with a cooler packed with food because there are no gas stations or fast food places on earth that offer fresh, whole foods.

You have to figure out what habits stem from your own choices and what habits have been made by other people's choices. You have attachments to certain foods and you need to reassess them. Do you always go out to eat with your family or friends?

What if you start new traditions? Anything that is learned can be unlearned. It's just going to take a bit more effort and time.

Eating at Different Times

One of the greatest tips I've ever received is to not eat at the same times every day. Why? Like anything, if you eat out of habit, downing the same bowl of oatmeal at 7:00 a.m. or consuming that 10:00 a.m. protein shake, even if you're not even hungry, your brain will come to expect fuel at that exact time, no matter what. You're not even allowed to check in with yourself to see if you're *really* hungry, to see if the physical demands of today are different from yesterday. If you had a good breakfast and have been sitting for three straight hours, do you honestly need that giant burrito? Did you perform a physical activity that warrants a protein shake? Do you ever need a protein shake, or are you just conditioned to think you need one? Do you really need an entire bowl of oatmeal, or are you just conditioned to eat that specific amount? Experiment to see how you feel with more or less food, at different times of the day. Start using your body's own clock to adjust when you eat and how much.

Regaining Efficiency

It's no surprise we are eating the wrong foods. Since man was created, there have been many conflicting views about hunter-gatherer societies and what we are "supposed" to eat today. While eating movements have surfaced (paleo, vegan, Mediterranean, etc.) all based on the way our ancestors ate, much of this research is futile, as many populations ate what they could hunt or find. When food was available, they ate. When food was scarce, they didn't eat. Whether we were omnivores (eating animals and plants) or even frugivores (eating all fruits, some veggies, seeds, and sprouts), most of us will never live in just one box. We won't belong to a single label. There are too many choices, too many options, and way too many temptations. How could you ever be satisfied with just fruit? Or just meat?

Let's take fruit, for instance. In the paleo community (or people who are on other diets) fruit is often discussed in a negative capacity. But fruit is the perfect food. It's low in calories, high in nutrients, full of water, and here's the best part—the part that people try to refute again and again—fruit does not require an insulin response to break it down. I repeat, there is no insulin response from fructose. But we've all heard that certain fruits are bad, that they are too high in sugar, etc. Do you feel bad after you eat fruit? Do you get constipated when you eat fruit? No. Start paying attention to your own choices and not what others are doing.

In a conversation about cancer and science, Johnny Cooke joked, "You want to stave off cancer? Starve yourself, and you won't get sick." We had a good laugh about it, because to say something like that to the general public would obviously not be smart. While he was clearly joking, there is irrefutable scientific evidence with the link to the *amounts* we eat and the toxins in our systems. When we constantly eat, eat, eat and store, store, store without enough exercise and proper elimination, we become toxic.

As I've mentioned before, it's not always what we eat that's the problem. For instance, you may think, "This is a pesticide. I ingested it, so it will do damage." However, it's not that simple. It's not the toxin, but the reaction in our bodies to that damage. It's our own toxins we produce to get rid of the invader that causes the undue stress and over time, preventing our bodies from being efficient.

Combine Exercise with Calorie Restriction

So, how do we get efficient again? The first step is to exercise at high effort levels (at a high enough level that will cause a major damage response) post-glycogen depletion. This will sound off the alarm in our bodies to get to work.

Proper nutrition is the second key. This means not eating in excess but not severely undereating either. You have to find the right balance where you can get your body efficient and function optimally. It's different for everyone.

The reality of digestion is that it does elicit a low-level damage response in the body, so the more you eat, regardless of what it is, the more you elicit that low-level damage response. This is why caloric restriction, especially in terms of detoxifying the body, matters so much. This is also why plant-based eating is so healthy. It's not because meat is intrinsically "bad," but that it's almost impossible to overconsume calories on vegetables and plant-based foods. It's like you are unknowingly fasting while bringing in nutrients.

Your reduced calories combined with exercise can make your body very efficient with minimal effort.

Smaller, Nutrient-Packed Meals

If you've ever eaten a giant meal and are still hungry, you might wonder why. Quite simply? Lack of nutrients. Our bodies are smart. They will keep signaling they are hungry until we give them adequate nutrition in the form of nutrient-dense food. Make this a rule: The majority of what you eat should come from quality whole foods.

Lack of nutrients has everything to do with hunger. If you've ever craved high-sugar foods or are truly hungry after a big meal, chances are the meal you just ate was high in simple carbs and lacking quality nutrients.

Remember: If you aren't constantly taxing the system, it has time to heal, repair, and do its job. Eating a smaller, nutrient-rich meal versus a large, nutritionally devoid meal is better for you, your waistline, and your brain. This is why fruit is such a superfood, as it's easy to digest and extremely cleansing to our bodies.

Dining out has vastly skewed what we think proper portion sizes should be. We are so used to the "bigger is better" mentality, that we think proper portions are too small. A proper single serving usually fits in the palm of your hand! This is why that giant salad can work wonders into tricking your body into getting the calories it needs with the ability to chew on substantial fare (versus scarfing down a burger or burrito).

Decisions for Baby

So, what does all of this have to do with detoxing and readying yourself for a baby? Everything. Unfortunately, many women don't have a positive relationship with food. We diet; we underconsume or overconsume; we skip important meals (even when we are hungry); we down too many drinks; and then we bring all of this baggage into our pregnancies. Add hormonal changes and weight gain on top of that, and you are setting yourself up for a lifetime of frustration, dieting stops and starts, and most likely, teaching your kids to be unhealthy too. How many obese kids have you seen who have fit parents? This is your moment to press the restart button, *before* you conceive.

Most women overeat when they are pregnant, gorging on food until they feel sick. While cravings can be very real, the actual extra amount you need is truly equivalent to a giant smoothie.

That's it: 250–450 calories does not constitute much, and spreading those calories out with a little extra teaspoon of nut butter here, a banana or a larger serving of quinoa there, is all you need to grow a healthy, happy baby.

It's important to make sure these calories come from quality sources, however, and not an extra serving of ice cream.

Trust me: Getting a handle on what you feed your body before you're pregnant, during pregnancy, and post-pregnancy can have a positive effect on your hormones, your mental state of mind, and your life post-partum. Banish those baby blues with a solid diet. Yes, even when you can't exercise for six weeks, you can lose the baby weight. It's all about knowledge.

Studies estimate we make about 227 food-related choices per day.

Budgeting What You Eat

You've probably heard the phrase "falling off the wagon." When it comes to creating a lasting, healthy attitude and relationship with and toward food, we all need backup plans to get back on track.

A realistic strategy is to start "budgeting" for your food the same way you would budget money. When presented with the following risks of falling off the food wagon, here's how to recover, and quickly.

Going to a Birthday Party

Whether it's an adult's birthday party or a child's, abstaining from cake or bringing your own food can seem rude and can make you or your child feel like the odd one out. Make sure you eat something nutritious and substantial before you attend, so you are not hungry. Drinking a full glass of water or two before you leave will help as well. Once there, if you want to abstain from chips, cookies, and cake, simply say you just ate and aren't eating sweets this week. People usually won't push when questioned. You have to be unafraid of feeling like the odd one out. Do you care more about what others think about you not being "one of the pack" or about your health? Who says you have to eat cake at a birthday party?

Be social without a drink or food in your hand. If you are the one who's always glued to the snack bowl, arrive late and say you can only stay for a few minutes. Get your social time in, and hit the road. If coming late isn't an option, ask the host if you can bring a dish for yourself (or for others to try). Leave the anxiety at home and realize that no one is bullying you into eating crappy food. Change the birthday party habits.

Going Out with Friends

Try suggesting activities that aren't surrounded by food. If you and your gals always go out to a restaurant or to a wine bar, suggest something different instead. What's something you've never done? Is there a physical activity you've always wanted to try? From indulging in spa treatments to visiting museums, use your city as a tourist stomping ground and make it a point to do something new every time you get together.

Going to a Movie

I've joked recently that I can't take my daughter anywhere without packing snacks, water, almond milk, etc. As if she can't go a solid two hours without food! It's the same with movies. This is where that sneaky "breaking your routines" habit comes in. Even if we have lunch or dinner beforehand, the smell of popcorn is often too tempting to pass up. Do what my hubby and I do. Pack some healthy snacks and sneak them in. We often pack homemade popcorn, grapes, or even no-bake energy bites. Yes, it's against the rules, but save your money and stash snacks in a big purse. The average movie theater popcorn is drowned in butter, fat, sodium, and calories. Ever had an extralarge bag of popcorn you split with someone? You're looking to ingest around 1,120 calories, 72 grams of fat, over 1,200 milligrams of sodium, and 120 grams of carbs!

Going Out to a Nice Dinner

If you're used to indulging during a nice night out, you can still enjoy your fine dining experience and eat well. If you know the restaurant, it's a good idea to call ahead to give the chef specific guidelines. Always ask to go light on the salt and oil. Double up on veggies whenever possible. Avoid cheeses, heavy sauces, and ask how meat (if you're eating it) is prepared. Stick to clear alcohols, like gin, and avoid mixers.

Going Out of Town or on Vacation

Traveling can often feel like sabotage for those who pay special attention to their exercise and dietary habits. Using your own body weight for workouts and staying active (even if you're relaxing) is one strategy. Taking advantage of fresh ingredients, local markets, and what's in season can help with healthy food options. If there are no healthy options, stop at a grocery store and stock up on healthy bars, nuts, seeds, and fruit. If you have to eat out every meal, ask a lot of questions and stick to foods that seem the least processed. On vacation and you really don't care? Up your exercise (whether it's swimming, paddle boarding, biking, etc.) and try to curb late-night eating.

Going to a Bar

I've always been the person who doesn't drink. Or, if I do, I'll have one and then be tipsy. (Yes, I'm a lightweight.) I honestly just don't like the way alcohol makes me feel, which to some is unfathomable. But, I've been to numerous bars in my life and only ordered water. If this isn't you, stick to clear alcohol, red wine, or even ciders, which are usually gluten-free (but higher in alcohol content). A hard and fast rule: For every cocktail you consume, drink a full glass of water. No exceptions. Yes, you will have to pee a lot, but it will keep you from feeling terrible or taxing your body. You can also take an activated charcoal before or after you drink to absorb the alcohol in your system. (This is a great remedy for stomach bugs as well.)

Hunger After a Meal

What about if going out isn't the problem? What if, like me, you have a habit of eating after dinner, or you eat too much at dinner? What if you honestly feel like you are genuinely hungry? As I sometimes do with my toddler, distract yourself. Distraction is key. Eat a decent amount at dinner, and then brush your teeth. Drink a big glass of water. Go for a nice walk. Stretch. Get ready for the next day. Write. Do yoga. Retrain your brain not to be focused on food or what comes after dinner. Signal to your body that you are done for the day. Period. Let your digestive system rest. If this doesn't work, take the seesaw approach. Have one "good" day, then one "normal" day. Just go back and forth for the entire week.

Unfortunately, our habits at home are the hardest to break. They might come and go in cycles. You might be successful one day and not the next (hence, the seesaw). Good old-fashioned mind control and thinking about what you're doing *for* your body is the only way to be successful. A few nights of not eating after dinner will not only benefit your waistline, but should help you sleep better and wake up with more energy, as your body's had more time to rest and heal.

At the end of the day, it's not about being perfect or never indulging. It's about making your slipups the exception rather than the rule. Can you eat "well" 80 percent of the time? What about 50 percent? Be realistic and see where you can improve.

Deciphering Your Hunger Pangs

Feeling hunger pangs? What you're feeling may actually be a signal for something other than hunger. Ask yourself the following questions:

AM I THIRSTY? Often, when we don't drink enough water, we can think we're hungry when we are actually just thirsty. Are you consistent with your water intake?

AM I TIRED? Being tired can stimulate hunger and make us eat more, when really, we just need a nice nap.

AM I STRESSED? We've all been there. Stress eating is a very real thing. Assess what's happening, and if it is stress, call a friend, write an email, go for a walk, or hit the gym.

The Story on Your Skin

Our skin tells the story of everything that's going on in our bodies, and oftentimes, you will notice one side of your body might be worse than the other.

Ever since I was a child, I've had a "thing" with the left side of my body. When I was born, I had a very noticeable birthmark on my left arm; my left hip caused my foot to turn out as I began to walk; my left tear duct was clogged; and later, I developed an arachnoid cyst on the left parietal lobe of my brain that required brain surgery.

I was an active, stubborn child who had a raging temper. I firmly believe the food my family ate (which often came from a box, can, or package) and the amount I ate had a lot to do with the way I acted and felt. At the same time, I put an unreasonable amount of pressure on myself to succeed. I was a perfectionist, an overachiever—physcially, mentally, and everywhere else. I suffered from painful, cystic acne as a teen, never paying attention to the harsh chemicals I was using, the immense amount of stress I was under, or the foods that I ate. I used to down a box of Wheat Thins without even blinking, jars of peanut butter, boxes of cereal, veggie burgers, one-pound baked potatoes followed by dessert followed by a giant 500-calorie smoothie at Smoothie King. I had a voracious appetite because my body craved *nutrition*, not calories.

Through college and long after, I experienced a slew of health problems I couldn't pinpoint. I decided to get off birth control (after prolonged use) and my hair began to fall out. I went to a few doctors, who suggested I might have polycystic ovary syndrome (PCOS). Or that, perhaps, my thyroid wasn't functioning or maybe I had too much testosterone. Nothing was definitive.

As I watched my hair disappear and my hormones go crazy, I was desperate for a cure. I never paid attention to the source of the meat I ate at the time, or the fact that I was in a very miserable relationship. I spent most of my twenties longing for something else, and once I made the decision to change my life, *every single* health issue went away. My hair grew long. No more hormone problems. No PCOS. No high testosterone.

Then, after giving birth, I noticed that the right side of my face began to break out, as well as my back and shoulders. Obviously, my skin was trying to tell me something, but what? Was it a coincidence that I wasn't sleeping, that I was so stressed about money I could barely get out of bed? That we had tried to put eggs and salmon back in our diets so our toddler could try them? That we had made a move to a place that was hotter than the surface of the sun?

If you're not using something on the outside of your skin that's irritating you, you have to look internally. When there are blockages in your body, whether from environmental toxins or food, they don't have anywhere to go. Everything we feel, do, think, see, and absorb manifests in our bodies. If we don't have a way "out," then we suffer. If you're "backed up," those toxins will find a way to escape, even if it's through your skin.

But the good news? You can fix it. You can pinpoint what's happening and eat foods to help get things moving along. You can address the constant battle of stress by asking yourself how you are thinking and feeling, how you can calm down, and how you can react to less-than-stellar situations.

The Five Rules to Detox

On your path to cleansing, there are going to be obstacles. Stressors. Emergencies. Breakdowns. Birthday parties. That's just life. There are things we associate with having a good time, such as consuming a million calories and too many cocktails.

But no matter what your day is like or how hard cleansing feels, there are five rules to live by—not just when you are in detoxification mode, but at any time.

1. DRINK WATER. This seems like the most boring and obvious rule there is, but it's one of the easiest ways to flush the system and rid your body of unwanted toxins. I can't tell you how many days I've been exhausted or my skin starts to flare up, and I realized (shockingly) that I'd only had a glass or two of water! This used to seem impossible, as water is almost all I drink. But, as the hours fly be in a haze of deadlines and computer screens, I fall prey.

2. EAT FRUIT. Some people shy away from fruit because of the sugar, but here's a fact: Fruit is the most easily digestible food there is. Our bodies can process and expel fruit in minimal time, more than vegetables, nuts, seeds, grains, and especially protein. Fruit is one of the only foods that can be eaten raw, doesn't need refrigeration, and comes in a variety or flavors and textures. Fruit doesn't need to be boiled, baked, or heated. Eat it first thing on an empty stomach to reap the most benefits.

3. EAT GREENS. If it's green, eat it. Because most people don't enjoy eating veggies raw (unless they are in a salad), juice your veggies or blend them to get a huge dose of calcium, iron, magnesium, and protein. This is one of the simplest ways to get those important micronutrients, especially if you don't like veggies. Hunt down anything that has chlorophyll and consume.

4. GET RID OF WASTE. Waste can accumulate in the body over years, resulting in stagnant, impacted matter that can manifest into disease. Remember: What doesn't get eliminated accumulates in the body. So, no matter what—eliminate daily. (I am not suggesting a laxative; rather, eating fiber-rich foods, drinking enough water, and as much as possible, not eating meat, dairy, or an abundance of grains. If you do need help, however, enemas and colonics are an option, as well as certain herbs prescribed by professionals.)

We are made to eat our food and then expel it, quickly digesting the food, absorbing the nutrients, and moving on to our next meal. Unfortunately, we don't eat easily digestible foods on a daily basis and often combine hard-to-digest foods with almost every meal. Focusing on easily digestible whole foods can make a life-changing difference in your diet and life. But waste doesn't stop with what you eat. Every day, it's important to get rid of the other waste—whether that's emotional, mental, or physical. If you are someone who eats the right foods or moves their bodies in the right way, congratulations. But are you happy? Do you stress over the smallest things? Does one bad moment ruin your entire day? Are you considered "type A" or high strung? You have to find ways to get rid of this "emotional waste" now, especially before a baby comes and your sanity is ripped from you before you can even blink.

5. EAT ONE FOOD AT A TIME. If the thought of eating clean overwhelms you, focus on one food at a time. Eat a bowl of one fruit in the morning, have just a salad for lunch, and enjoy just pasta for dinner. Think simply. Whenever you reach for a snack, stop worrying about combining foods to get the right amount of protein. Reach for one food. Eat it, digest it, and if you're still hungry, reach for something else.

The Skinny

While there are numerous tips and tricks you can implement into your daily life and different reasons for choosing or not choosing to do "well" on any given day, the most important thing is to adhere to the goals you set for yourself. It is the *most* important thing to success: the follow-through. Set the goals—just as you would in work, sports, love, etc.—and achieve them. Get up tomorrow, set new goals, and achieve those. Be kind to yourself. Listen to yourself.

When we watch these weight loss shows, we see people who are sequestered in an environment where they eat, sleep, and breathe exercise; where they are given the tools to eat right and are allowed to discuss past traumatic issues that have caused them to pack on 150 extra pounds. But, this is not real life. When the duties and responsibilities of daily life are taken away, almost any one of us could reach great feats. We could reach our true potential. But most of us aren't given that opportunity. We don't live up to our full potential. We think small, but dream big. What's that instance, quote, book, or experience that's going to shake you awake and make you realize that you're missing it? That while you are stressed about the phone bill or the fact that your husband forgot to put the toilet seat down *again*, time is moving, and we are growing older, and there's no guarantee for anyone?

We have our health. We have our lives as we've created them. We have choices. Choose health. Choose to get rid of the junk in your life: emotional, physical, and mental.

Use the tips in this chapter for your detox and every day after. Arm yourself with knowledge to pass along to your children, especially when they start making their own food and lifestyle choices. Give them (and yourself) the best foundation you possibly can.

Because when everyone else is thinking and talking about and doing one thing, you have to be willing to choose a different path. Ask the different questions. Start a new conversation about food and what works for you.

CHAPTER SEVEN

The Detox Before the Detox

Many people go into detoxes full-force, binging on greasy food and alcohol the night before and quitting everything cold turkey the day of, which makes cleansing much worse. It also makes it much easier to give up when you experience detoxifying symptoms from the foods and substances you love.

The state of your health is nothing more than a culmination of lifelong habits, which can feel almost impossible to break. Can you *really* have dinner without dessert? A fun night out on the town without cocktails?

Enjoyment is important, but most of us have had more enjoyment than we can possibly handle when it comes to food and alcohol. When you are readying yourself for a baby, taking care of your body is where you should get your enjoyment. How healthy can you make your baby's home? In our baby craze, we rush about, purchasing clothes and cribs and making sure the house is organized and baby-proofed when we bring a baby home...yet what about its internal home? Shouldn't this be the first priority?

Preparing your body for detoxification is the first step in readying yourself for pregnancy. The "detox before the detox" can help ease powerful detoxification symptoms once you do cleanse (no one wants to feel like they have the flu!). Omitting certain trigger foods, allergens, alcohol, and other substances *ten days to two weeks* prior to cleansing is optimal for an easy cleansing transition and lasting health. They say it takes twenty-one days to make or break a habit, but you'd be shocked at how easy it is to kick even your toughest vices after just ten days.

The best part? Many of the items we will omit before the detox are foods/substances that are not recommended once pregnant. Allowing your body time to acclimate without sugar or caffeine is better than quitting cold turkey once you find out you're with child. Let me tell you: Suddenly saying good-bye to your daily pot of ridiculously strong coffee does not a happy camper make.

By easing yourself into this program and figuring out which foods are your triggers, which foods have been making you feel terrible for years, and which foods make you feel incredible, you can head into your pregnancy with renewed knowledge, health, and energy for a thriving pregnancy, delivery, and foray into motherhood.

Pull the Trigger

We all have our trigger foods. For me, it's chocolate or anything sweet after dinner. No matter how well I've eaten, after dinner, like clockwork, I want a piece of dark chocolate, a huge batch of almond butter chocolate chip cookies, or a bowl of nondairy ice cream. Why? Pure habit. I associate these foods with my daughter as I let her lick the vegan cookie dough batter. She takes small bites, runs a lap around the house and comes back asking, "More? More, please?" I associate dessert with curling on the couch with my husband; our eyes glassy as we dunk fat, fresh-baked cookies into our icy almond milk while watching bad reality television at the end of an interminably long day.

Dessert is my reward for a productive day, a hard day, a great day, a so-so day. I feel entitled. I *earned* that sugar!

It's taken me well over thirty years to realize this isn't the way to lasting health. While a dessert here and there won't hurt, taxing my body with sugar at the end of *every* meal wreaks havoc on my pancreas, liver, and skin. It affects my joints and my sleep, and makes me feel like I have a hangover the next day. The bottom line? Sugar is a powerful drug that I don't need in my daily life. I *know* this. But knowledge and execution are two different things.

But I am also realistic. Will I go without dessert for the rest of my life? No. But, I can go in cycles. I pay attention to my habits, and if I indulge, I pay the price the next day, when I struggle through the morning in my sugar coma. I have realized it's not just "indulging" I'm doing; at this point in my life, it's damage. Once a week? No problem. If healthy, our bodies can usually assimilate nutrients and expel toxins from our system with minimal effort. But, the more your poor food choices become daily habits, the easier it is for toxins to build and manifest into disease.

It's imperative that you figure out what your triggers are *before* your cleanse. Ask yourself:

- What foods do I turn to when I'm stressed?
- What foods do I reach for when out with friends?
- What foods do I eat the most? (Take inventory of breakfast, lunch, dinner, snacks, and drinks.)

- If I splurge, what do I splurge on?
- What's my favorite food?
- What food(s) can I absolutely not live without?

Write your answers to these questions and use the tips/swaps in this chapter to go shopping. The following chart is a useful guide when going shopping:

Trigger	Swap
Alcohol	Kombucha
Caffeine	Herbal tea
Sugar	Sucanat, date sugar, molasses, raw honey
Beef	Bison, emu
Raw Sushi	Cooked salmon
Peanuts	Almonds, Brazil nuts, walnuts
Conventional soy products	Fermented soy
Chicken eggs	Duck eggs
Cow's milk	Nondairy milks
Refined grains	Whole grains
Butter	Coconut oil

Do some quick Internet searches for healthier homemade options, use the recipes in this book, or purchase a healthier alternative. If you really love candy, research that candy. Read all about what goes into it and its effects on your body. Educating yourself can often make you realize that you have just been eating that food out of habit. There are so many different types of food just waiting to be eaten that are derived from whole foods and will make you feel great.

When you're shopping for new finds, follow one rule: Read the ingredient list. Purchase items with ingredient lists you can pronounce and understand.

If You Love Alcohol, Try Kombucha

For some, giving up alcohol can be one of the hardest parts of any detoxification program (or pregnancy). First, you must understand how alcohol affects the body. According to Brown University Health Education, the liver can process one ounce of liquor (or one standard drink) in one hour. If you consume more than this, your system becomes saturated, and the additional alcohol will accumulate in the blood and body tissues until it can be metabolized.

Your body works incredibly hard to break down alcohol, but it stays in your system, and if pregnant, passes to the fetus. Ridding your body of any alcohol prior to pregnancy is key for a healthy baby.

Kombucha can be a natural antidote to alcohol (though it still contains a trace amount of alcohol). Kombucha, or fermented tea, contains a plethora of enzymes, probiotics, vitamins, and minerals. This ancient drink has been around for over 2,000 years. Despite its Asian roots, kombucha has come a long way and has become an American staple. It totes an infinite list of benefits for the body, the gut, and overall health. According to a YumUniverse.com article, studies show that kombucha repairs damage caused by environmental pollutants, lowers levels of toxins, is potent in detoxifying the liver and preventing chemical-driven liver damage, prevents cancer, and that its consumption even limits the effect of radiation. It's also been known to reduce symptoms of fibromyalgia, depression, anxiety, and kidney stones, as well as treating arthritis, alkalizing the body, improving eyesight, increasing metabolism, stimulating and improving digestion, rebuilding connective tissue, alleviating constipation, relieving headaches and migraines, boosting energy, improving mood, clearing complexions, speeding the healing of ulcers, relieving symptoms of PMS, and lowering glucose levels.

It comes in a variety of flavors and can be bubbly like champagne. For beer lovers, this is a great swap.

If You Love Caffeine, Try Herbal Tea

We all love our coffee, but caffeine, whether from a soda or a latte, steals energy that your body just doesn't have. What does that mean? You will crash...eventually. You begin to need more and more just to feel the same jolt of energy. While coffee has gotten a good (and bad) reputation over the years, allowing your body a break from caffeine is imperative to let your digestive system work on its own without that extra kick, as well as giving your adrenals a rest.

And trust me, ladies. Herbal tea might become your new best friend while trying to curb morning sickness (hello, ginger!) or taking the edge off at night. If herbal tea sounds drab, try finding an apothecary in your town and get a special brew made just for you. Don't have an apothecary nearby? Head to your nearest grocery store and hit the tea aisle. If there's an ailment, there's a tea to cure it. Look for pregnancy teas and enjoy yours with a bit of honey and lemon to let the soothing begin. Not ready to kick coffee yet? Start mixing regular coffee with decaf to lessen the strength. Gradually change to decaf coffee then transition to black tea, green tea, and then herbals when you're ready.

If You Love Sugar, Try Sucanat, Date Sugar, Molasses, or Raw Honey

I'm sure you've heard the news that sugar is bad. Not all sugars are created equally, however. We should all aim to stay away from adding any processed or white sugars to our foods or drinks. According to *Forbes*, Americans consume 135 pounds of sugar *per person* per year. That equates to 22 teaspoons per adult *per day* and 32 teaspoons per day for children!

While sugar wreaks havoc on the body, there are safer forms that can be ingested in moderation. Sucanat (natural sugar cane), date sugar (sugar spun from dates), raw honey (which totes numerous medicinal properties), or even molasses can be swapped in place of your white table sugar. Because sugar is incredibly addictive, cutting back is the first step in a healthy detox plan. Eliminating added sugars and then focusing on getting your sugars from natural sources, such as fruits, is a step in the right direction. You will notice clearer skin, more energy, and better sleep quality when you cut back on sugar.

If You Love Beef, Try Emu or Bison

While red meat is high in saturated fat and cholesterol, some people feel like they actually need red meat once in a while, which is fine. But for the purposes of detoxification, we want to refrain from any hard-to-digest meats, and red meat tops the list. If you are dying for a steak in the future, opt for emu or bison, both of which contain a high amount of protein and healthy fats. Emu (an Australian bird) is heart healthy, while low in fat, cholesterol, and calories. It's high in protein, iron, zinc, phosphorus, magnesium, and vitamin C. It contains more protein per serving than beef and is also higher in iron. Bison are not "handled" as much as cows and are therefore left alone to munch on grass (not in feedlots). They are usually not subjected to drugs, chemicals, or hormones. Like emu, they are also higher in protein and iron than beef, but lower in calories and cholesterol. A perfect alternative to red meat.

If You Love Raw Sushi, Try Cooked Salmon

Who doesn't love sushi? If eating sushi is part of your life, giving up fish might seem next to impossible while detoxing or pregnant. However, mercury in our fish supply has become a huge problem.

According to Catherine Guthrie's article "Fertility Diet," mercury is toxic to a developing fetus and can linger in a woman's bloodstream for more than a year.

The good news is that not all fish contain the same amount of mercury. Furthermore, the US Food and Drug Administration (FDA) says that women trying to conceive can safely eat up to twelve ounces (roughly two entrées) a week of low-mercury fish, such as shrimp, light tuna, salmon, or catfish.

What's on the "avoid" list? The list changes often, but the FDA suggests avoiding canned albacore (white) tuna, as well as fresh or frozen swordfish, tilefish, king mackerel, tuna steaks, shark, orange roughy, Spanish mackerel, marlin, and grouper because they have the highest mercury levels.

Be sure to do your research and talk to the fishmongers at your local markets. While there are numerous types of fish that register lower on the mercury scale, eating cold-water fatty fish, such as salmon, still ranks high in terms of omega-3 fatty acids, which your body needs for the brain and developing fetus. Cook up some salmon and make your own rolls (with cooked, low-mercury fish) at home to munch on when the sushi craving strikes.

Get Your Omega-3!

Since our bodies don't make omega-3s, it's vital to get them from outside sources. Omega-3s have been known to help with a baby's eye and brain development, as well as slashing some serious risks for pregnancy (pre-term labor, preeclampsia, depression, etc.). Numerous plant-based sources of omega-3s include walnuts, flaxseeds, chia seeds, and quinoa. If you don't like the taste of fish, try high-quality fish oil supplements or plant-based supplements sourced from algae.

If You Love Peanuts, Try Almonds, Brazil Nuts, or Walnuts

Peanuts are one of the dirtiest crops around (and one of the biggest allergens to adults and children). Contrary to popular belief, peanuts are not nuts—they're legumes. Finding quality organic peanuts is next to impossible, and the health risks often outweigh the benefits. Swap with raw organic almond butter (which has the same amount of protein), Brazil nuts (high in selenium), or walnuts (high in omegas). Soaking almonds releases all those yummy nutrients as well. Brazil nuts and walnuts cannot be sprouted. Aim for a handful or two tablespoons per day.

If You Love Conventional Soy Products, Try Fermented Soy

Soy is another dirty crop and has gotten an awful rap throughout the years. Conventional soy should *never* be consumed, especially while pregnant. Finding fermented sources, such as natto, miso, or organic tempeh, are acceptable choices, if eaten in moderation. Fermented soy is easier to digest and can even promote bone and heart health. High in calcium and a complete protein, toss fermented soy products into a stir-fry for an easy, nutritious meal.

If You Love Chicken Eggs, Try Duck Eggs

If you love eggs and grab any old carton, think again. Even if your carton says "cage free" or "organic," that doesn't mean much. Often, chickens are packed so tightly (even when cage free), they have no room to relieve themselves and are often sick and will die, festering with disease, among other live chickens. Duck eggs, while more expensive, contain more protein and have a richer taste than chicken eggs. They are also alkaline forming and stay fresher longer due to their thicker shell.

They also contain more omega-3s. While higher in cholesterol, they contain six times the vitamin D of chicken eggs and twice the vitamin A. Even better? Most people who are allergic to chicken eggs do not have a duck egg allergy. If duck eggs aren't an option, find local eggs that are humanely raised. This will not only ensure better nutrients and quality control, but an exceptional taste as well. Cutting back on eggs pre-pregnancy and throughout pregnancy is recommended, as eggs are one of the largest allergens to infants and children (most of whom outgrow this allergy).

If You Love Cow's Milk, Try Nondairy Milk

Why shouldn't you drink milk? Quite simply, because you're not a cow. Humans are made to consume human milk, just as cows are made to consume cow's milk. It's really as simple as that. We are the only species to consume other species' milk. It's no wonder so many people cannot digest milk and have such a hard time with dairy in general. If you aren't a fan of nondairy alternatives, search for organic goat milk, which compares in chemical balance most closely to human breast milk (especially when feeding toddlers). When searching for nondairy alternatives, always opt for organic selections and read the ingredient list! Many nondairy milks contain gums, gels, and carageenan, all of which should not be consumed, especially while detoxing. Always search for milks that don't have added sugars and are devoid of these common additives.

Can't find one you like? Making your own nondairy milk at home is easy and delicious. Simply purchase the type of nut or seed you wish to "drink," and use the ratio of one cup of nuts or seeds to two to three cups of water. Blend in a high-speed blender, adding in one or two dates (optional), cinnamon (optional), or even a probiotic, and then strain with a nut milk bag or sieve. (If you opt for hemp milk, there's no need to strain.) Store in the refrigerator for three to four days.

Sample Food Swaps

Make at least one healthy swap with every meal. Do not opt for low-fat, fat-free, or sugar-free substitutes of the same processed foods. What would a healthy day of swaps look like?

Meal	Usual Food	Try Instead
BREAKFAST	Egg McMuffin and coffee	Sprouted English muffin with almond butter and herbal tea
SNACK	Muffin	Green smoothie
LUNCH	Pasta and bread	Brown rice pasta, red sauce with veggies, and a small green salad
SNACK	Candy bar	Fruit and nuts
DINNER	Burger and fries	Veggie burger and sweet potato fries

But remember, it's all about baby steps. You want to make sure the changes you make stick, so make your swaps incrementally over stages.

Trigger	Stage 1 Swap	Stage 2 Swap	Stage 3 Swap
BREAD	Whole wheat bread	Sprouted wheat bread	Raw bread/ Manna
CHIPS	Pita chips	Rice chips	Kale chips
COOKIES	Gluten-free cookies	Vegan cookies	Raw cookies
PASTA	Brown rice pasta	Mung bean pasta	Zucchini noodles
BURGERS	Bison burgers	Black bean burgers	Raw nuts and seeds
FRENCH FRIES	Baked steak fries	Baked butternut squash	Baked sweet potato
WHITE RICE	Brown rice	Millet	Sprouted quinoa
CHEESE	Organic cheese	Daiya cheese	Nut cheese
ICE CREAM	Goat milk	Almonds	Banana

If You Love Refined Grains, Try Whole Grains

Refined grains, found in processed foods such as cookies, chips, crackers, and white bread can be some of the hardest to kick, especially our beloved bread. Walk into any grocery store and the chips, cookies, and bread choices can seem infinite (and inviting). While there are many "gluten-free," "made with organic ingredients," and "low-fat" items on the market, most are just loaded with nutritionally devoid ingredients. If it comes in a bag, skip it, and opt for healthy grains or veggies instead. If you can't kick your processed food habit just yet, read every ingredient. Short ingredient lists without added oils, salt, and sugar are preferred. If you love bread, search for organic, sprouted varieties, which are easier to digest. Remember, a short ingredient list is key.

Ready to try a grain or pseudograin (seed)? Quinoa, teff, buckwheat, millet, and amaranth are at the top of the heap. Most contain complete protein, vitamins, minerals, low to no fat and no sugar. Try out different swaps based on what your taste buds enjoy.

If You Love Butter, Try Unrefined Coconut Oil

People say butter makes everything better! We've got one better than butter: coconut oil. Not only is coconut oil one of the most multipurpose products on the market, its antimicrobial, antifungal, antiviral, antioxidant, and anti-inflammatory properties can help you heal both internally and externally. From diaper rash to conditioner, coconut oil's uses are vast. Though it is high in saturated fat, our bodies do not like to store it as fat since coconut oil is a medium-chain triglyceride. What does this mean? Our bodies like to use it for energy instead. With a low melting point, it tastes deliciously decadent spread on sprouted toast or used in place of butter in sauces. Simply melt it to a liquid and use it in place of other oils in both cooking and baking.

The Skinny

Whatever your vices, there are healthy options to replace them. Examine your diet to pinpoint the biggest culprits. Things to absolutely cut out during this phase: fast food, sodas, chips, alcohol, bread, cigarettes, heavy meats, dairy, and cookies. If you want to detox, you should start here. Take stock of what's in your kitchen, your pantry, and your refrigerator. Look at the foods you love the most and choose a healthy alternative. Detoxing before you detox is often the hardest but most beneficial part to get your body used to what is to come!

CHAPTER EIGHT

The DBYE Foods

While detoxing focuses on what we can get *out* of the body versus what we are putting into the body, it also introduces foods that enhance health, cleanse the system, and boost fertility odds. All foods listed in this chapter are those that you should and can eat. Studies have shown these foods increase fertility and cleanse the body, which is exactly what you want to do. Notice that most of these foods are plant-based. As I stated earlier: You do not have to give up meat (especially after this plan), but taking a break from digesting proteins and dairy is beneficial to effectively cleanse and thoroughly detox the system. Surprisingly, you might find you have more energy and are just as satisfied. Listen to your body. If you want meat, try restricting it to dinner and aim for at least three plant-based days per week.

Most of the foods in this chapter are rich in color and pack a nutrient-dense punch. The list is extensive. Choose from foods you like, and every week, swap out those same tried-and-true foods for new ones. Variety is just as important as what you eat.

Budget-Friendly Tips

Purchasing too much food can be overwhelming, not to mention wasteful. To cut back on grocery costs, do a quick inventory at home of the staple items you already have or need. Think about good-for-you items that perform double duty (e.g., apple cider vinegar can be used in salad dressings and with nondairy milk to make "buttermilk"; cacao can be mixed with avocado for a chocolate pudding or thrown into a smoothie; tahini can be used for hummus, sauces, or even when baking). Look at what foods you eat the most and what can be purchased to add flavor. Think about fresh herbs and spices.

Once you have your staple list, aim to purchase just a few fruits and veggies each week. You can even pick one color of the rainbow for each week. For instance, this week, you are only going to buy green produce; next week, purple, then red, yellow, orange, etc. Each week, only pick two or three fruits, three veggies, one nut, one seed, and one grain. This makes your grocery list easy and less expensive. Think about the multipurpose functions of each food and how they might fit together for various meals. If you purchase quinoa, broccoli, tomatoes, and avocado, for instance, you can make great stir-fries for the week and then throw the leftovers onto some lettuce for a salad. You can use leftover quinoa for a breakfast porridge. Garbanzo beans can be roasted or blended to make hummus. Chia seeds can be tossed into smoothies or mixed with almond milk for a delicious chia pudding.

Each week, make a new list of produce, seeds, nuts, and grains you want to try. Don't get in the habit of just plucking from the same groups of foods over and over again. You won't get all those vitamins and minerals you need if you are eating the same handful of foods. Branch out. Maybe even focus on eating what's in season (which can often be cheaper). If you already eat the fruits and veggies that are in season, you can design your meals around what's local or in your CSA, versus thinking up recipes all the time.

Eat for Fertility

All of the foods listed below will detoxify the body and also boost fertility. Foods in the protein category are more for beginners and those who still want to include meat in their lifestyles. Experiment with foods in each category to see how you feel. The following list has been adapted from Steven Pratt's *SuperFoods Rx for Pregnancy*.

Fruits (fresh, dried, and freeze-dried)

- Apples
- Apricots
- Avocados
- Bananas
- Blackberries
- Blueberries
- Boysenberries
- Cherries
- Cranberries
- Currants
- Goji berries
- Grapes
- Grapefruits
- Kiwis
- Kumquats
- Lemons
- Limes
- Mangos
- Nectarines
- Oranges
- Papayas
- Peaches
- Pears
- Persimmons
- Pineapples
- Plums
- Pomegranates
- Raspberries
- Strawberries
- Tangelos
- Tangerines
- Tomatoes

Vegetables/Fresh Herbs

- Artichokes
- Arugula
- Asparagus
- Bell peppers
- Bok choy
- Broccoli
- Brussels sprouts
- Butternut squash
- Cabbage
- Carrots
- Cauliflower
- Celery
- Chives
- Cilantro
- Collard greens
- Daikon
- Eggplant
- Garlic
- Kale
- Kohlrabi
- Leeks
- Liverwort
- Mustard greens
- Onions
- Parsley
- Pumpkins
- Romaine lettuce
- Rutabagas
- Scallions
- Seaweed
- Shallots
- Spinach
- Sweet potatoes
- Swiss chard
- Turnips
- Turnip greens
- Watercress
- Wasabi

Nuts/Seeds

- Almonds
- Cashews
- Chia seeds
- Flaxseeds (ground)
- Hazelnuts
- Hemp seeds
- Macadamia nuts
- Peanuts
- Pecans
- Pine nuts
- Pistachios
- Pumpkin seeds
- Quinoa
- Sachi inchi seeds (SaviSeeds)
- Sesame seeds
- Sunflower seeds
- Tahini
- Walnuts

Legumes/Beans

- Garbanzo beans
- Great northern beans
- Green beans
- Green peas
- Kidney beans
- Lentils
- Lima beans
- Mung beans
- Navy beans
- Pinto beans
- Split peas
- Sugar snap peas

Grains

- Amaranth
- Barley
- Brown rice
- Buckwheat
- Couscous
- Oat bran
- Oats
- Kamut
- Millet
- Rye
- Spelt
- Wheat germ
- Wild rice

Meat-Based Proteins

- Chicken breast, skinless
- Clams
- Crab
- Halibut (Alaskan/Northern)
- Herring
- Lobster
- Mackerel
- Mussels
- Oysters
- Salmon, wild-caught
- Sardines
- Trout
- Turkey breast, skinless

Dairy

- Greek yogurt
- Kefir
- Raw whole milk

Oils

- Coconut oil
- Grapeseed oil
- Extra-virgin olive oil

Soy (Organic)
- Miso
- Natto
- Tempeh

Teas
- Green tea
- Black tea
- Oolong tea
- White tea
- Rooibos tea

Superfoods

I'm hesitant to use the word "superfood," as I feel this word isn't always honest in its meaning or delivery. However, for the purposes of this list, superfood just means foods that serve dual purposes in their ability to cleanse and heal. There are countless foods like this in the world (including many standard fruits and vegetables). You do not have to include these in your diet, but feel free to experiment to see if you notice any health gains.

ACAI BERRY: This berry comes from a palm tree and is best known as a little "cancer fighter" due to its ability to destroy up to 86 percent of leukemia cells in vitro. In addition, it helps weight loss and is a stem cell producer. Even better? It contains 19 amino acids, is a source of omega-3 fatty acids, and is incredibly rich in antioxidants.

AVOCADO OIL: We all know that avocados contain healthy fats. Use this hearty oil in dressings or marinades to help increase healthy high-density lipoprotein (HDL) cholesterol levels. The oil can even be used to soothe skin inflammation or as a moisturizer for hair!

BEET JUICE: If you look at a beet's rich color, you know it's packed full of antioxidants. Beets can help enhance athletic performance, promote brain health, and even lower blood pressure. Juice or blend beets at home and enjoy alone or with other fruits and veggies.

APPLE CIDER VINEGAR: Apple cider vinegar has some serious medicinal properties. A spoonful of apple cider vinegar first thing in the morning can improve digestion, return the body to an alkaline state, clear up heartburn, cleanse the skin, and promote circulatory health. Use it in dressings or baking, or consume it on its own.

BELUGA LENTILS: Because of their rich, black color, these little cancer fighters battle inflammation and slash heart disease risks. Swap with your regular lentils and use instead of a meat-based protein. Stir-fries and soups with beluga lentils make easy, tasty dishes. Note: Many people have a hard time digesting lentils, even if they are sprouted. Use your judgment. You do not have to include lentils in your diet (or any bean or grain for that matter) if you can't properly digest them.

BLACK GARLIC: Its dark color attests to black garlic's high zinc content. This naturally fermented food improves nutrient availability while maintaining its natural antibiotic properties and has even been thought to promote a longer life. Can't find black garlic? Regular garlic works wonders as well. Because it is a natural antibiotic, the next time you have a yeast infection, skip the Monistat and insert a clove of garlic instead. (Yes, really.) Inserted overnight, you can cure yeast with just one clove.

CHLORELLA: This algae is a complete protein containing all B vitamins, vitamins C and E, and a huge dose of iron. It helps immune function, improves digestion, and accelerates healing as well. This chlorophyll-rich food can detoxify the liver and brain while boosting immunity. It can also help arm you against harmful viruses or bacteria. A bonus? Chlorella contains 65 percent protein, which is almost the highest of any food!

FERMENTED VEGGIES: Since fermented vegetables are made with live cultures, you are getting a healthy dose of probiotics, which is vital to a healthy gut. While we always think of bacteria as a negative, fermented veggies deliver millions of friendly bacteria to the digestive tract, which can help aid immunity, digestive wellness, and even increase your ability to heal from an injury.

MACA: An Incan superfood, this root is instrumental in boosting immunity and increasing energy and libido. It is well known for its ability to help enhance endurance and strength. It contains vital B vitamins and vitamin C, and can even help increase fertility. Purchase in powder form and add a tablespoon to smoothies.

MORINGA: It might sound like a birth control device, but this African and Asian plant helps with blood building and digestion. While helping to reduce aging and inflammation, it's also a complete protein source. It contains eighteen amino acids as well as B vitamins, vitamin E, and traces of vitamin D2. Vitamin B12, which can be hard to get if you're plant-based, is abundant in moringa. Much of the plant is edible. The leaves are rich in protein, vitamin A, vitamin B, vitamin C, and minerals. In only half a teaspoon (of its powder form), you can get over 100 percent of your daily B12 requirements! It's also high in calcium, copper, iron, magnesium, phosphorous, potassium, zinc, and antioxidants. Search for the seed, leaves, or powder at your local health food store.

SAVISEEDS: These little powerhouses contain seventeen times more omega-3s than salmon and nine grams of complete protein. Also known as sachi inchi seeds, they can be found in most health food stores for blending or tossing in smoothies.

SEA VEGETABLES: More commonly known as seaweed, these veggies are the most nutrient-dense around. Containing ten times the calcium in cow's milk, they are a complete protein source, a natural source of electrolytes, and an endurance enhancer. Kelp, dulse, arame, and kombu are just a few sea veggie options. If you don't like the taste of sea veggies, search for the flakes or powders and add them to your smoothies or juices.

SPIRULINA: With the antioxidant equivalent of seven servings of vegetables, this powerhouse algae contains vitamin K, vitamin A, iron, chlorophyll, and more protein than beef per serving! Toss a teaspoon of the powder in your smoothie for a dose of nutrients in the morning, or mix with avocado for a delicious spread. Want some double duty? Spirulina works great as a pop of color for eye shadow as well.

SPROUTS: Sprouts contain an abundance of vitamins and minerals and are easily thrown on top of salads or sandwiches. A great source of free-form amino acids, they help with detoxification and have enzymes that help aid in rejuvenation. They are also rich in nutrients, making them one of the best nutritional powerhouses you can eat. Make sure you always purchase fresh sprouts (they should never be slimy). Or, make your own at home by soaking and then waiting for "tails" to grow on your grains, seeds, or legumes. Eat within a day or two of purchasing (or sprouting).

ZA'ATAR: This spice blend of sesame seeds, salt, sumac seeds, and thyme can actually decrease your risk of food-borne illnesses. Use in savory dishes or purchase all ingredients separately and make your own blend!

Spice It Up

If you think all herbs and spices are created equal, think again. If your spices of choice are salt, pepper, and sometimes paprika (if you're feeling wild), you're missing out on the detoxification properties of numerous spices and herbs.

When we detox, we focus on eliminating toxins, but this can sometimes flush out the good bacteria as well. In addition to eating fermented foods or taking a good-quality probiotic supplement, consuming the following ten herbs and spices can help "wring out" your organs to aid in the detoxification process. Many of them can be added directly to food, taken on their own, or even found in pill or oil format for a more potent dosage. Eating raw? Don't be afraid to add to smoothies or shakes.

CARDAMOM: A plant of the ginger family. Attacks harmful bacteria and expels it from the body. Can also act as a natural antidepressant.

CAYENNE PEPPER: Helps the body lose weight, speed up metabolism, improve digestion, and eliminate waste.

CINNAMON: Helps detox the body, control blood sugar, treat yeast infections, alleviate stomach bugs, reduce irritable bowel syndrome (IBS) symptoms, ease arthritis, and is antimicrobial and antibacterial. Take alone or add to a detox shake or smoothie for best benefits.

CUMIN: Helps digestion run properly to expel toxins from the body.

GINGER: Cleanses and helps the body absorb nutrients and minerals. Good for digestion and reduces detox symptoms, such as flatulence and bloating.

HORSERADISH: Helps liver screen out carcinogenic substances and other toxins. Helps with sinus infections and urinary tract infections (UTIs), and is a natural cancer fighter.

OREGANO/OREGANO OIL: Cures upper-respiratory infections, slashes cancer risks, boosts immunity, is anti-inflammatory, is antimicrobial, and helps rid the body of parasites. Add fresh or dried oregano to food or purchase pure oregano oil and dilute with water to ingest directly. (This can even be rubbed on the soles of a child's foot to help rid them of colds.)

ROSEMARY: Rich in antioxidants. Helps all systems function properly. Helps with toothaches, eczema, and joint and muscle pain.

SAFFRON: Big boost to internal organs. Helps bladder and kidneys, beneficial to the liver. Helps the body naturally detox.

TURMERIC: Helps the liver function, totes anticancer properties, is anti-inflammatory, reduces oxidative damage, boosts brain function, lowers heart disease risk, reduces arthritis, and reduces depression.

A Note about Sourcing

So, you've purchased healthy foods—this should be enough, right? Do you know where all that food comes from? From young Thai coconuts being sprayed with formaldehyde, to seaweed that's toxic after the Japanese nuclear meltdown, to crops that are grown near farms that attract chemical runoff from traffic or nearby construction, to high arsenic levels with rice, the items you throw into your shopping cart could use a little research on your part. This is why going to local farmers' markets or attending markets that have strict rules about sourcing is important and can be educational for you and your family regarding different farming practices and regulations.

It may seem like a headache, but it all goes hand in hand with educating yourself so you can help educate your children and make eating a fun, informative process.

CHAPTER NINE

The DBYE Program

Before you launch full force into the DBYE program, it's important to understand what to do and what not to do when it comes to detoxifying the body. Depending on what category you fall into in "Determining Your Detox Plan" (page 57), detoxifying can take a toll on the body as it expels toxins and flushes bacteria, parasites, and even viruses.

If you've ever had the flu or a stomach bug, then you know what it's like to detoxify. Though unpleasant, the body works very hard to give the digestive system a break and expel any invaders from your body. While detoxifying willingly usually isn't this intense (unless you are supremely sick), you can feel a plethora of symptoms, such as exhaustion, mood swings, headaches, body aches, and diarrhea. Because of this, it's important to stay hydrated and not take on vigorous exercise if you are doing a cleanse for the first time or experience strong symptoms. Those who are used to eating healthy may notice only positive side effects, such as better sleep, a more active colon, and more energy.

The Do's

1. EAT LIGHT TO HEAVY. What does this mean? Often, we start our days with starches and proteins. If you love eggs and toast, you know what I'm talking about. Because proteins take the longest of any food to digest, if your body can't break down that food quickly, anything you eat after can get "clogged" and putrefy in the gut. Put a sandwich on top of that at lunch, followed by a heavy dinner, and you are asking for rotting food and a sluggish colon. But there's an easy fix. Since fruit is the easiest food to digest, followed by greens, starches, and then proteins, reorder the foods you eat in that manner. Start your day out with a delicious green smoothie (or fruit), followed by a starch. Lunch can be a giant salad (still keeping it light) and dinner can be reserved for those proteins and veggies. Take this order into consideration as much as you can: fruits, greens, starches, proteins.

2. GET PLENTY OF SLEEP. Sleep is just as important as the food you eat or the water you drink. In the last decade, with technological advances and entrepreneurship, sleep is more disturbed than ever. Work is no longer limited to the office. We can work late into the night from the comfort of our bedrooms. If you are detoxing your body, try detoxing your mind as well. Limit your screen time to an hour before bed and try to calm your mind. Refrain from eating at least two hours before bed to help with sleep. Sleep is your body's time to rest and repair itself. While eight hours is not feasible for every person, try going to bed a half-hour to an hour earlier than usual at night and wake up without an alarm clock whenever possible. Even if this equates to just a little more sleep, it helps. It's good to note that the most critical and restorative sleep for the nervous system occurs between the hours of 10:00 p.m. and 2:00 a.m.

3. STAY HYDRATED. Try to drink eight to eleven glasses of liquid a day, preferably water. While all food contains water, and most fruits and veggies contain around 80–90 percent water, listen to your body. If you are thirsty, drink! You cannot properly detox without water to flush the toxins from the body, so aiming to drink water first thing in the morning and throughout the day is important.

4. EXERCISE. Staying active throughout the day allows toxins to move through the system. If exercise turns your stomach, start thinking of the term "exercise" in a different way. What activities do you enjoy? Dancing, cleaning, walking? These are all forms of exercise. If you can, try to spend the majority of your day moving instead of sitting. If you have an office job, see if you can rig a standing desk or set a timer on your watch or phone to alert you to move throughout the day. Do some triceps dips, squats, push-ups, and gentle stretches to open up the chest and back. Walk around the block and about the office, or take the stairs instead of the elevator. Want to go a step further? Sit on a stability ball at your desk or stash a jump rope and resistance band in a desk drawer for some quick, functional fitness. Start looking for daily ways to get more exercise. When parking at the store, choose the farthest spot parking spot you can. Walk as much as possible. Go hiking. Ride a bike. Put music on at home and have a dance party. Just move. Detoxifying the body is as much about eating as it is about getting healthier and stronger from the inside out. Fitness is a huge component of this cleanse and should be a priority in your life. If your budget allows, opt for a few massages during your cleanse, as well, to keep the lymphatic system moving and allowing those toxins an "exit" point in the body. How? Movement of the body, such as through exercise, pushes lymph through the system. Massage also pushes lymph through the system and can be extremely beneficial to reduce inflammation post-workout. For those who are interested, this is a time to research colonics as well.

5. EAT WHEN YOU WANT TO. Eating just three times per day allows the digestive system a break, especially if you are a chronic snacker. When you are constantly eating—even if they are small meals—it's hard to clean out the body and give the system a chance to rest, recover, and heal. If you generally eat three meals per day, plus two snacks, check in and see if you are really hungry or if you're just conditioned to eat at that specific time. If you eat at the same time every single day, it's easy to "think" it's time to eat.

This is especially true for mornings. We hear that we have to eat breakfast as soon as we wake up to jump-start the metabolism. Now, if you are hungry when you get up, by all means, eat. But when we sleep, we rest, repair, and heal. Once you start eating again with breakfast, you are back to digesting your food instead of healing the body. This is why it's so important to give the body something light and nutritious in the morning instead of something heavy and starchy. So, wait until you're really hungry to eat.

If you are an athlete or are incredibly active, however, a little more thought needs to go into your meal planning, especially if you are training in the morning. After fasting all night, your body does need energy to perform. Many people get up and exercise without eating anything. If you're going for an easy walk around the block or doing light cardio, this is fine. But if you're asking your body to do more work or training for a sport, it doesn't have energy supplied from food to steal from, so it must pull from your body's own energy supply. Eating something small, like a banana or a few dates should sustain most forty-five-minute to one-hour workouts.

Going longer? Mix some coconut oil and lemon juice in with those dates for little energy bites that will keep you sustained for hours.

---

6. LISTEN TO YOUR BODY. This might seem like a fairly obvious tip, but it's a tried-and-true method. When you eat something, pay attention to how you feel directly after, thirty minutes after, and an hour after. Do you have energy? Are you suddenly exhausted? Do you feel like taking a giant nap? This is a great exercise to do beyond your cleanse to figure out what you should and shouldn't be eating—especially while pregnant. If you can figure out now what foods give you energy and which steal energy, it will be easier to decipher when pregnant and contending with hormones and food cravings.

While you are detoxing, it's easy to experience sugar or caffeine withdrawals, but you might figure out there's something else you've been eating for years that has been making you feel awful. That cold that never seems to go away? Perhaps it's the cream in your coffee. The sandwich you eat a few times a week? It might be contributing to that cough or itchy eyes. Because food is handled much differently than it was in our parents' and grandparents' generations, we have to pay attention to the quality of our food and all the many processes it goes through. The fewer processes, the better. By eating mostly whole foods, you will rapidly see which foods are contributing to your health and which have been making you feel less than healthy.

7. BUY A BLENDER. A good-quality blender is one of the best investments you can make for your health. Not only can you make smoothies, soups, dips, or sauces, you can easily make juices by blending produce and then straining with a nut milk bag or cheesecloth for a delicious cold-pressed smoothie. A good blender is vital for pregnancy and making your own baby food (which is so much quicker, fresher, and easier than you think) in the future. Research different brands to see what's best, and don't skimp on quality! Drinking a chunky green smoothie versus a perfectly blended smoothie can make all the difference in sticking to a healthy food plan.

8. FOLLOW THE "FOOD COMBINING" RULES 50 PERCENT OF THE TIME. A definite school of thought and research backs up the principle that when it comes to digesting your food, you can omit a lot of the bloating, gas, and discomfort by paying attention to what foods you eat together or apart. (However, people with insulin resistance or diabetes should not adhere to these principles.) Even if you haven't heard of food combining, you've probably heard that proteins and starches don't mix. Why? When the body breaks down proteins (meat, dairy, eggs, fish, seeds, nuts, protein powders, etc.), it requires an acidic environment to properly break them down, and they take the longest to digest. Starches (bread, crackers, pasta, grains, and starchy vegetables) require an alkaline environment to break down and digest. So, when you combine your burger and fries, you are asking your body to do two separate things. The acids and alkalinity end up neutralizing each other, which taxes the body, leaving you exhausted. The differing environments don't allow for proper digestion or assimilation of nutrients.

Upon first cleansing, give the body a prime opportunity to digest appropriate foods at appropriate times to help jump-start quick elimination, boost energy, and rid the body of toxins in a much more timely fashion. While food combining isn't mandatory for a successful cleanse, I would suggest heeding cues from Natalia Rose, nutritionist and author of *Raw Food Life Force Energy*. Below she notes five general categories and rules for food combining:

- Starches: bread, pasta, whole grains, potatoes, legumes, cooked corn
- Fleshes: all animal flesh, eggs, and cheese
- Nuts and seeds
- Dried fruit
- Fresh fruit

The food-combining rules?

- Starches should only be combined with other starches, as well as all raw and cooked vegetables.

- Fleshes should only be consumed with other fleshes, all raw veggies, and all cooked non-starch vegetables.

- Nuts should only be eaten with other nuts, seeds, dried fruits, bananas, and raw veggies.

- Dried fruits combine with other dried fruits, avocados, bananas, nuts, and all raw veggies. Fresh fruit should only be eaten alone on an empty stomach.

Cheat Sheet on Food Combining

(from Kimberly Snyder, author of *The Beauty Detox Diet*)

- Starches DO mix with vegetables.
- Proteins DO mix with vegetables.
- Proteins and starches DO NOT mix.
- Different starches DO mix.
- Different proteins DO NOT mix.

- Fats DO NOT mix well with protein; pair moderately.
- Fats DO mix with starches.
- Fruits should be eaten on an empty stomach.
- Fruit DOES mix with raw greens (except melons).

If this principle makes your head spin, don't worry. It's something to keep in mind if you want to try it and can accelerate cleansing if rapid detox is your main goal. Not for you? Stick to the gentler beginner detox (page 121). The choice is yours.

The Don'ts

1. DON'T SKIP MEALS. While intermittent fasting is practiced by some (as mentioned at the beginning of this book), it is not advised to skip meals, especially while doing a whole-foods cleanse. If you've never eaten breakfast, you might think it's

not important to start now. Wrong. If you are notorious for eating one meal a day, it's time to aim for three. Forget the snacks and just focus on balanced nutrition through breakfast, lunch, and dinner. A smoothie in the morning, a large salad for lunch, and a soup or something heavier at night. Make a schedule for your food, just as you'd make a schedule for work. We are trying to jump-start our systems, get rid of waste, and rev our metabolisms in preparation for baby. Remember *why* you are doing this. You want to be as prepared as possible so you can be successful.

2. DON'T EAT PROCESSED FOODS. The entire point of a whole-foods detox is to avoid those muffins, cookies, chips, etc. (This doesn't mean forever. Just while cleansing.) If you literally cannot fathom going without processed food, get your baking trays out and make some healthier snacks at home. Grinding your own flours from almonds or oats to make muffins or pancakes at home is certainly healthier than grabbing that muffin at a café. If you are really "all in," however, attempt to go this short period without processed food to allow your body a chance at true recovery. A great exercise is to track your eating for a few days before your detox and count how many foods you eat that are processed. This extends to condiments, drinks, and anything that's been through a processing plant. Once you start taking inventory of the foods you eat, look at what's in your house. What's in a box, can, or bag? Taking inventory can be a bit shocking, but also motivating in terms of how good you can feel by even switching a few of those processed foods with fresh foods.

3. DON'T BINGE AT NIGHT. If eating at night gives you serious trouble, whether from actual hunger or habit, make sure you are eating a very balanced, nutrient-dense meal at dinner that will satiate you throughout the night. Maybe this is when you can have your heavier proteins or starches (remember not to combine these two, if possible, while cleansing), or if you're eating lighter, up your intake so you are full of fiber and are therefore full. Making a cup of hot tea or drinking a few glasses of water can help flush the system and keep the body full at night as well. Think of night as your chance to heal and repair, especially while you sleep. If you can eat dinner several hours before bed, even better. You never want to eat and then go directly to sleep. Your body will be forced to digest your food instead of repairing your body while you sleep.

4. DON'T FORGET WATER. Yes, this is on the "do" list as well, because it's just that important! It's so easy to go through your day and not even get a few glasses of water in. You get busy; you're not thirsty, etc. Keep a glass bottle (or two) with you at all times to remind you to drink. Set a reminder every hour on your phone to drink water. This is one of the absolute most important parts of your cleanse! Make it a priority.

5. DON'T DIET — DETOX! I'VE SAID IT BEFORE, BUT IF YOU GO INTO THIS CLEANSE THINKING OF IT AS A DIET, YOU WON'T LAST. Think about wringing out those organs, expelling waste, and making a healthy environment for your baby. For once, eating has a purpose. Getting a handle on your nutrition and how your body should really feel prior to conception will make pregnancy a wonderful, enlightening experience.

Quick Health Tips for Everyone

USE AVOCADO IN PLACE OF DAIRY. Cut and freeze avocado and blend with banana, cacao, and nondairy milk for a creamy smoothie. Mix with nondairy yogurt, herbs, and spices for a yogurt sauce, or even blend avocado with garlic, basil, and lemon juice for a creamy pasta sauce.

MAKE A GOOD SAUCE. A big bowl of veggies can seem super boring unless you dress it up with a good sauce. While sauces can pack a ton of fat and calories, they're a great opportunity for throwing antioxidant-rich superfoods into your meal. Opt for avocado, tahini, nut, seed, or coconut oil–based sauces. Make a big batch and store in a mason jar for up to a week.

SWAP YOUR MORNING GRAIN. Instead of making oats yet again, opt for quinoa, buckwheat, millet, or teff in its place. Rotate weekly and vary your toppings.

MAKE FAUX CHEESE. Nailing a good nut cheese or faux cheese is definitely an art. Some of the best sauces for mac and cheese include lemon juice, cashews, coconut oil, and nutritional yeast, but many people (myself included) stay away from cashews, as the double shell surrounding the raw cashew contains a resin that can create significant skin rashes and can be toxic when ingested. Many people have extreme sensitivities to cashews and prefer to use other nuts.

Swapping the nuts with seeds in your go-to recipes is a great way to try new tastes. (Once I took out cashews, I realized just how often I was eating them. From desserts to sauces, they were in everything!) Opt for sesame seeds or hemp seeds to see how they take on the flavor. Not afraid of nuts? Soaked almonds or organic walnuts blended with herbs, spices, nutritional yeast, and lemon make great creamy sauces or pesto.

MAKE VEGGIES THE STAR PLAYER AT EVERY MEAL. Thanks to society, the "star" in most of our meals is animal protein. Rather than ordering a chicken breast and getting a side of vegetables, ask for what vegetables are on the menu and devise your meal around those. Really want protein? Add a side of beans or piece of fish. If a restaurant isn't open to doing that, simply supersize your veggie order and nix the unhealthy additions. When you're at home, do the same. Got a wonderful butternut squash or cauliflower? Make this the center of your meal. Roast that veggie, blend into a soup, or toss with other greens and top with a delicious sauce.

ADD STRONG HERBS. Herbs add flavor without guilt and offer an array of nutritional benefits. Grating ginger into a sauce or tossing fresh cilantro, garlic, or parsley adds freshness to any dish and often satisfies the taste buds without blowing your caloric budget.

Sample Daily Meal Plan for Your Detox

So, what does a typical day look like in the midst of a whole-foods cleanse? Recall your detox type from "Determining Your Detox Plan" (page 57) and look below at a sample day on your plan. Don't like what you see? This is just an example of what you should be eating. Hate bananas? Switch them out with another organic fruit. This is about making a detoxification plan work *for* you, not against you. But, be open to trying foods you may have stayed away from in the past. Often, you can find a preparation of fruits and veggies that you actually enjoy. If all else fails, that morning green smoothie will work wonders to get your daily intake of veggies.

	Beginner	Intermediate	Advanced
BREAKFAST	Chocolate Almond Butter Shake (page 173)	Green Dream Shake (page 171)	Ginger tea, followed by Detox Green Juice (page 171)
MORNING SNACK	Trail mix	Kale chips with hummus	Raw crackers with hummus
LUNCH	Brown rice, black bean, and avocado bowl	One-pound salad with pumpkin seeds/homemade dressing	Giant raw "noodle" salad
AFTERNOON SNACK (OPTIONAL)	Raw Chia Pudding (page 170)	Hemp protein shake	Power Greens Shake (page 172)
DINNER	Red sauce with veggies over quinoa pasta	Soba noodles with creamy sauce, veggies	Large salad with raw tacos

Tips for Success

It's important to set yourself up for a successful cleanse. Tell family members, coworkers, and friends what you're doing and why. You can even see if a friend wants to do it with you. Make sure to have the following in place before starting:

CLEAN OUT YOUR KITCHEN. You wouldn't believe how easy it is to lose those fresh veggies and fruits to plastic bags at the back of your refrigerator. Fresh foods get lost, especially if you go to the store without cleaning out your refrigerator, pantry, or taking stock of what you have at home first. So sift through your cupboards, pantries, and refrigerator to see what you can get rid of and what you can use with healthy dishes. If fruits or vegetables don't need to be refrigerated, placing the four or five you want to eat that day on the counter is a great way to remind yourself to eat what's in front of you (or pack them for work).

MAKE A GROCERY LIST. You have to figure out what type of shopper you are. Do you do better if you shop for just a few days, or do you need to shop for the entire week? Do you like knowing exactly what you are going to make, or do you like throwing together dishes from the items you buy? If you're like me, you might make one or two meals at the beginning of the week, and by Wednesday, you're ready for a night out. Know this about yourself and plan accordingly. If you want to eat out on Wednesday, you can still stick to your plan. Try a new place or frequent a vegan or plant-based restaurant in your area, which will often have healthier options. Know what meals you are going to make with the items that you purchase. Don't just buy food and have no idea what you're going to do with it. Having taken inventory of your fridge and pantry before you go to the store, you should be able to throw easy meals together in no time.

EAT EVERYTHING. Obviously, you don't need to eat *everything*, but when you start running low on produce, take inventory of what you have left. Can you juice or blend the leftovers? Can you throw those veggies together for a quick soup or stir-fry? Do you consistently buy berries or greens that go to waste? Freeze them! Every year, thousands of pounds of food are wasted. See what you can do with those odds and ends scattered about. Some of my favorite meals are ones that my husband will throw together with our "five ingredients or less" rule. Choose five random ingredients and set a timer for twenty minutes. See what you can whip up.

BUDGET FOR YOUR SCREWUPS. What aren't you willing to do? If you know for a fact that you are going to have a dessert or a glass of wine, then "budget" (page 70) for it. Plan a healthier day after your "cheat," or make sure to plan a quick activity after you indulge. If you eat a giant scoop of ice cream while on this cleanse, don't just sit there—move! That's why it's vital to take this a single meal at a time. Remember, this is not deprivation or a diet. Just as you would go to the doctor for a checkup, this is a way to do maintenance yourself. Once you get all the junk out, it's easier and easier to do little "spot cleanses" over time. Managing your expectations with reality is vital to lasting success. So, know yourself and plan to pick yourself up when you screw up. This is especially important before pregnancy, as when you give in to cravings during pregnancy, it's not as easy to get up and go for a run.

The Skinny

As with pregnancy, this detox is a journey. There's no perfect weight, perfect cleanse, or exact amount of toxins to expel that will ensure you have the best pregnancy, a healthy delivery, and a baby who doesn't cry or throw tantrums. Life is messy. Motherhood is messy. Parenting is loud. Eating well all the time is hard. Through all of this, especially during your cleanse, try to find the balance, whether you're tired, moody, annoyed, or stressed. Try to make better decisions today than you did yesterday, so that they become a habit before you get pregnant and have a baby.

Once these habits are firmly rooted in place, getting up four or five times per night won't want to make you run for that pot of coffee and loaded bagel. You'll know better. You'll know what it *really* feels like to feel better and have energy, and how you can continuously feel and look great by paying attention to what you put in and on your body.

Let the cleansing begin.

CHAPTER TEN

Detox, Detox, Detox!

You are primed and ready to detox your body, mind, and life. You are ready to stop thinking about what you don't want to look and feel like, and instead start focusing on who you want to be. It is finally time to clear out the junk, slash health issues, and get your body ready for baby.

On the following pages are three detoxes: beginner, intermediate, and advanced. Recall your detox type from "Determining Your Detox Plan" (page 57) and use this as a guide for your specific program. You can use these suggestions as general guidelines or follow the step-by-step rules to eliminate toxins and cleanse the body. You can also pick and choose recipes or eating plans from each cleanse (or use them as a ladder as you make progress), since they are all complementary in nature.

Remember this isn't about following the plan to a tee, but learning to shift your habits and mindset and creating concrete ways to get back on track when life (or a baby!) gets in the way.

Toggling Calories

As mentioned at the start of this program, the option to toggle calories is available and can be one of the absolute most vital components to this cleanse. What does this mean? Toggling calories is reducing your baseline caloric intake by 25 percent for two to three days within a three-week time period (while maintaining your baseline caloric intake the remainder of the days). This intermittent fasting focuses on *temporarily* decreasing your calories without resetting your baseline caloric intake.

By purposefully reducing caloric intake by 25 percent for two to three days every twenty-one days, you will jump-start the system and allow all the benefits of detox without *actually* fasting. Because this is infrequent, you won't adapt to this brief calorie reduction.

So, for example, say my baseline caloric intake is 1,800 calories per day. I know that this is the magic number I need where I won't gain weight and I won't lose weight. I can maintain my weight, even while working out, because my body is *used* to my activity level. I'm not starting a new sport or doing something out of the ordinary.

Now, for two or three days, I will reduce my calories by 25 percent, which will take me to 1,350 calories per day. If I were to maintain this number for two weeks, as you would do in most diets, my new baseline would become 1,350 calories, because my body would *adapt* to this new number. So, if I went back to that 1,800 mark, I would actually be in a surplus and *gain weight!* This is why diets do not work and people often end up gaining weight once they go off of them.

This is also why I would *only* reduce my calories for two or three days, before my body can adapt and generate a new baseline.

What's Your Baseline?

So, first things first. You must figure out your baseline. You can do this two ways. You can go and get your lab work done, which can be pricey, but can also give you the exact number you need. Here's another way:

1. Whether you are sedentary or active, do not embark on a new fitness regimen while trying to figure out your baseline calories. Figure out what your "normative" state is, whether you are sedentary or extremely active.

2. Figure out what your baseline caloric intake is where you do not gain weight and you do not lose weight. (Most of you might be there now; you just have to track your calories for a day or two.) You can find online sites that will calculate your age, height, weight, and workout intensity to come up with your baseline caloric intake. You can also calculate your basal metabolic rate (BMR) according to your height, weight, and age and multiply that by the appropriate activity level to find out your daily calorie needs. Check out www.bmi-calculator .net/bmr-calculator to calculate your baseline.

3. Once you have your number figured out, use the foods in this plan and count your calories to reduce them by 25 percent, either before you start your detox or once your detox has begun. Because you might initially be eating less during your detox, it's imperative that you don't drop your calories too drastically so as to drop your baseline. Again, this isn't about a diet. It's about cleansing the system, and there is a precision to the process. You can choose when and if you want to toggle your calories. Once you know your numbers and want to try, reduce the proper amount of calories for two or three days and then return to your baseline for at least twenty-one days. While counting calories is tedious, it is imperative when you are detoxing to make sure you are not overconsuming calories (because it's easy to do with the good stuff too).

Note: Toggling calories is definitely not recommended while pregnant or while nursing during the first year.

Good luck!

Beginner Detox

Let's get down to business. Are you going to magically wake up tomorrow and love kale? No. Are you going to have an easy time giving up sodas, caffeine, artificial sweeteners, alcohol, cheese, and fried food? Probably not. Oftentimes, seeing what is off limits can be harder than learning what you should be eating.

You probably know that eating healthy salads (not doused in bacon, cheese, and heavy dressings) and other whole foods are healthy. That fruits and vegetables are good for you. But you just can't manage to make that part of your daily life. You need guidelines to follow and a solid list of foods to eat. You need simple examples of how you can make healthy swaps, day by day. You need guidance, with a little bit of freedom.

For your cleanse, we are going to start with some general guidelines. It is especially important for you to start thinking about food in different terms. Remember: Think, don't decide. Once you have a handle on these guidelines, you can start to focus on what you *can* eat, rather than what you can't. Omitting the unhealthy foods gradually as well as taking your time transitioning should give you plenty of room to ease into a healthier way of eating. While eight weeks of healthier eating might seem interminable, if you break it down into daily or even weekly segments and are diligent about tracking your progress, you will gain momentum and get one step closer to a healthier body for pregnancy.

I recommend keeping a food log, as well as an energy log on how you feel daily (or even meal by meal) in order to track your symptoms and progress. Write yourself healthy reminders or have them texted to you by entering them at ohdont forget.com. Are you more of an accountability person? See if a friend wants to do this program with you, or post daily updates on your Facebook page so you can stay motivated and track your progress. Set non-food-related awards for yourself along the way. Seeing tangible results often fuels you to keep going, even when you feel like giving in and eating a cheeseburger.

Betsy Reed, holistic health coach and business consultant, has devised numerous cleanses for clients over the years, and has helped create the following general guidelines:

1. **ELIMINATE SODAS.** Replacing sodas with flavored sparkling waters, natural fruit juices, kombucha, or iced herbal teas will slash calories and decrease sugar intake. This will promote weight loss, lower blood sugar, and decrease yeast/candida growth. While it might seem hard at first, your body will quickly adapt to not consuming so much sugar. One soda has 37 grams of sugar—almost *nine* teaspoons! What happens to all that sugar? It wreaks havoc on the pancreas and is stored as fat. Period. There's not one positive thing about soda, other than its eating through battery acid. If it can clean steel, think about what it can do to your insides. Eliminate!

2. **SWAP BUTTER OR MARGARINE WITH OLIVE OR COCONUT OIL.** Swapping oils will promote weight loss and decrease risk of chronic diseases, such as hypertension and high blood pressure. Coconut oil has a plethora of health benefits and tastes surprisingly like butter. Our bodies don't like to store coconut oil as fat, so there is more chance of your body using it for fuel rather than storing it. With olive oil, always hunt for extra virgin and cook the oil over medium heat (or use in raw dishes).

3. **ADD COLD-WATER FISH.** Each week, replace two or three meat/processed meat dinners with cold-water fish. Which fish

are best? Wild salmon (not Atlantic), sardines, arctic char, Atlantic mackerel, sablefish, black cod, anchovies, oysters, rainbow trout, mussels, and Pacific halibut. Besides promoting a huge dose of omega-3s, replacing meat with fish will promote weight loss, decrease risk of chronic diseases, and improve digestion, which will lead to a better night's sleep.

4. SWAP WHITE RICE WITH BROWN OR BASMATI RICE. White foods are void of nutrients and are high on the glycemic index. Because they lack fiber, they often leave you feeling hungry. White foods can cause weight gain and increase risks for type 2 diabetes. Brown and basmati rice will provide more protein and fiber and maintain nutrients because they are not overprocessed. When purchasing brown rice, make sure you research which brands have the lowest arsenic levels.

5. REPLACE CRACKERS AND BREAD WITH WHOLE-GRAIN VERSIONS. Even when you find a box of crackers or a loaf of bread that says "made with whole grains," or "multigrain," that doesn't mean much. The label doesn't have to say how much of anything it includes, so take the safe bet and opt for whole grains, like rice or quinoa, instead of something that comes in a box. However, if you still want crackers or bread, search for those that are made with 100 percent whole grains and have as few ingredients as possible. Make it a rule that all the foods you buy have five ingredients or fewer. By purchasing foods with words you can pronounce and focusing on fiber and protein content, the body will break the food down more easily and assimilate the nutrients, which will help promote health and weight loss. Make sure to stay away from words like enriched, bleached, unbleached, or hydrogenated oils.

6. REPLACE MORNING CEREAL OR PASTRY WITH OATMEAL. Think oatmeal is just for kids? Think again! Oatmeal is high in fiber, extremely filling, and will not increase blood sugar. Plus, it will sustain you much longer throughout the morning and keep you full for hours. Not an oatmeal fan? Jazz it up with different berries, nut butters, raisins, and some raw honey. Or, opt for a quick, delicious, no-bake Overnight Oats (page 166) that takes one minute to prepare.

7. ELIMINATE PROCESSED/PASTEURIZED DAIRY AND USE ORGANIC/GRASS-FED DAIRY INSTEAD. After pasteurization, there is nothing good left in milk and cheese. All the enzymes are destroyed by heat. Select dairy products that come directly from the cow or goat and are grass fed. Even better, try a nondairy milk, such as hemp milk or almond milk. Always choose organic and read the labels to see what you're buying.

8. ADD MORE VEGGIES, EVEN IF THEY ARE PRE-CHOPPED OR FROZEN. Don't have time for washing and chopping veggies? Dump the cans and boxed food and use flash-frozen veggies instead. Flash-frozen veggies are washed and chopped and just need a quick steam or light boil (five minutes tops) to eat. Canned veggies are high in sodium because of preservatives added to extend their shelf life (which means more chemicals). Frozen veggies maintain almost all their nutrients and are tasty and delicious when lightly cooked to thaw. Throw into pasta sauces, soups, or use for easy ten-minute stir-fries.

9. STOP EATING CANNED FOODS. Who doesn't love a quick, easy meal? However, canned foods can lead to hypertension and sodium overload. Opt for Crockpot meals, where you can toss in meat, frozen veggies, and even your quinoa or brown rice. Set a timer before work and you're ready to eat when you get home. You can even add water with veggies to the pot and make a veggie stock for prepping other meals!

10. AVOID HIGH-FRUCTOSE CORN SYRUP (HFCS). Beware of high-fructose corn syrup. Our bodies do not recognize HFCS. Therefore, it digests quickly and goes straight to the blood. Why is this bad? When HFCS quickly passes to the liver, triglycerides and cholesterol develop, resulting in a fatty liver, which affects many Americans. HFCS also spikes insulin, which increases appetite, weight gain, the propensity for diabetes, etc. If you are going to eat processed foods, look for those containing real products, like cane sugar. Yes, real sugar in moderation is better for you than HFCS because your body actually recognizes it and can digest it. However, for the purposes of cleansing, we are trying to eliminate sugar, so use it sparingly.

Weeks 1 and 2: Omission Period

As previously discussed, it's time to focus on removing the trigger foods from your diet: wheat, soy, caffeine, alcohol, dairy, meat, eggs, sugar, peanuts, etc. By now, you should have identified what your trigger foods are and what you eat the most of in this category.

While the process for removing these foods is different for everyone, de-junking your kitchen is the first step to making sure you have all temptation out of your house. If you don't trust yourself to do it, enlist help from a friend or loved one (or even a health professional who specializes in nutrition and kitchen cleanouts). Read every label and ingredient to see where the preservatives, sugar, extra salt, and chemicals might be lurking. Donate any unwanted food so as not to waste it, and make a new grocery list for the week, making healthy swaps to have on hand at all times. If you like bread, find a sprouted variety. If you like cheese, opt for a healthier version (feta or nondairy). If you love fried chicken, opt for a roasted chicken. Dining out? Ask specific questions about what's in your food, how it's prepared, etc. Don't ever be afraid to ask! You can even call ahead and let the chef know your limitations. Most restaurants will be happy to accommodate your requests.

Next, allot a calorie budget for each meal. Try to stay under 400 calories for each meal, spaced four or five times throughout the day. While counting calories is not fun, in the beginning, holding yourself accountable to a number can help with overall success. It can also show you how much we tend to overeat and how much less we actually need, not only to thrive, but also to feel great. Fact: If you consume more than you expend, food gets stored. Period. It doesn't matter if all you're eating is lettuce—if you eat enough, it *will* be stored.

For every meal you eat, drink two glasses of water. One well before your meal and one after. Make this a habit to flush toxins from your system. Can't manage two glasses? Split the glass of water in half and drink half before and half after.

By the end of these two weeks, try to have at least three new healthy habits established. This period is more about elimination than incorporating healthier foods into your diet. We are trying to get your system used to going without its staple crutch foods.

Weeks 3 and 4: Transition Period

Every day, for every meal, you are going to choose *one* ingredient and swap it out with a better ingredient. For instance, if for breakfast you have cereal with milk, swap the regular milk for nondairy milk. The next time you have cereal, opt for a gluten-free version. Then, perhaps, try making your own granola or Overnight Oats (page 166). If you normally eat a burrito from Chipotle at lunch, swap guacamole for cheese, or forgo the tortilla and get a "bowl" instead. From the snacks you eat to the meals you make, choose one healthy swap per meal. Try to outdo yourself every day, perhaps trying a veggie you've never had, such as a fruit, a nut, or even a seed. Swap heavy dressings with apple cider vinegar and olive oil, dark chocolate for milk chocolate, almond butter instead of peanut butter, or Greek yogurt or nondairy yogurt for regular. This is your time to get smarter about what you put into your body. It's a time to aim for variety.

If eating out is your problem, start perusing some new dishes on the menu. Most menus offer healthier options these days and even share their nutritional facts on their menus and websites. Again, don't be afraid to ask questions to see how you can alter your favorite dishes to make them work with your plan. If you like fast food, too bad. Avoid! There are healthier chains out there, so if you need something fast, hit a chain that has at least heard of a vegetable. (McDonald's does not count.)

At the end of two weeks, you should not only feel better from having stayed away from these trigger foods, but having accustomed yourself to new tastes and options along the way.

Weeks 5 through 8: Clean Eating

For the purposes of your plan, we are sticking to basic options that can be obtained almost anywhere. Substitute anything you want, but use this as a guide. Eating three times per day with one snack in the afternoon is ideal.

Below is a one-week plan with three substitutes for each meal to try for the next month. You can choose the order in which you want to try these meals, using the idea of the simple swap to eat a plethora of foods and try new versions every week.

WEEK 1, DAY 1

BREAKFAST: Chocolate Almond Butter Shake

HOW TO MAKE IT: See recipe on page 173.

> **WEEK 2:** Swap the strawberries with blueberries, reduce to 1 teaspoon of almond butter.
>
> **WEEK 3:** Omit berries, swap almond butter for sunflower butter, and swap flaxseeds for hemp seeds.
>
> **WEEK 4:** Go back to week one's recipe. Toss in a handful of spinach and kale.

LUNCH: Burrito

HOW TO MAKE IT: Heat a sprouted or whole-grain wrap on the stove or in the oven. Boil 1 cup of water and add ½ cup of brown rice. Cook until fluffy. Rinse fresh-cooked or canned black beans. Heat them in a pan, then spoon them into the wrap. Add the brown rice, a sliced tomato, lettuce, mashed avocado (or guacamole), hummus, and salsa. Wrap and enjoy!

TIP: Search for gluten-free wraps or 100 percent whole wheat wraps.

> **WEEK 2:** Omit brown rice.

> **WEEK 3:** Omit wrap. Use only brown rice.

> **WEEK 4:** Drizzle tahini over the top of burrito bowl from week three.

AFTERNOON SNACK: Hummus and pita chips

HOW TO MAKE IT: Find an organic hummus and organic pita chips. You can make your own at home by baking tortillas and blending a can of rinsed garbanzo beans with lemon, tahini, sea salt, garlic, a little bit of water, and olive oil.

> **WEEKS 2, 3, AND 4:** Swap out pita chips with celery or carrots.

DINNER: Wild-caught salmon with baked sweet potato and steamed broccoli

HOW TO MAKE IT: Preheat oven to 350°F. Rub salmon with spices of your choice and place in a baking dish. Bake for 20–25 minutes (or to your liking). In the same oven, place small sweet potato on wire rack. Bake until soft in the middle, around 30–40 minutes. Rinse a small head of broccoli and steam on stovetop for 3–5 minutes, until slightly tender.

WEEKS 2, 3, AND 4: Rotate broccoli with kale, collards, cauliflower, or mustard greens and double up on the veggie portions to increase satiety.

WEEK 1, DAY 2

BREAKFAST: Pumpkin pie shake

HOW TO MAKE IT: Blend one frozen banana, ½ cup of pure canned pumpkin, ½ cup of frozen peaches, ¼ cup of chia seeds, three pitted dates, 1 cup of nondairy milk, and a pinch of cinnamon.

> **WEEK 2:** Omit the peaches.
>
> **WEEK 3:** Toss in a handful of romaine.
>
> **WEEK 4:** Keep your romaine from week three and omit two dates along with the peaches.

LUNCH: Pasta and salad

HOW TO MAKE IT: Opt for brown rice or quinoa pasta over regular pasta. Choose an organic red sauce with lower sodium or make your own with garlic, tomatoes, olive oil, and onions. Toss in some veggies or mushrooms with the sauce. This meal can be made in 10 minutes. Make one cup of dry pasta. Make a small side salad and consume it before the pasta.

> **WEEK 2:** Reduce to ½ cup of dry pasta and increase the veggies in the sauce by 1 cup.
>
> **WEEK 3:** Progressing from week two, sprinkle nutritional yeast over the sauce.
>
> **WEEK 4:** Try 1 to 2 cups zucchini or squash noodles (peeled with a spiralizer or a potato peeler) instead of regular pasta.

AFTERNOON SNACK: Brown rice cakes

HOW TO MAKE IT: Spread two brown rice cakes with 2 tablespoons of sunflower seed butter. Top with a handful of raisins, sesame seeds, and a drizzle of raw honey.

> **WEEK 2:** Omit one brown rice cake and 1 tablespoon of sunflower seed butter.

> **WEEK 3:** Progressing from week two, swap raisins with freshly sliced apple.

> **WEEK 4:** Progressing from week three, omit the honey.

DINNER: Quinoa salad with roasted chicken

HOW TO MAKE IT: Boil 1 cup of water and ½ cup of quinoa. Reduce heat, cover, and cook for 15–20 minutes. Chop up parsley, cilantro, and red pepper. Once quinoa is cooked, toss in herbs and pepper with a handful of raisins and sunflower seeds. In a separate cup, mix together 2 tablespoons of tahini, 1 tablespoon of organic Dijon mustard, and 1–2 tablespoons of water. Mix well and drizzle over quinoa. Shred roasted chicken and mix in with the quinoa salad.

> **TIPS:** Make sure the roasted chicken you get at the grocery store is organic. If you are trying to go meat-free, toss in some rinsed garbanzo beans instead.

> **WEEK 2:** Swap dates for raisins.

> **WEEK 3:** Swap sesame seeds for sunflower seeds.

> **WEEK 4:** Toss in spinach.

WEEK 1, DAY 3

BREAKFAST: Sprouted toast and toppings

HOW TO MAKE IT: Toast one piece of sprouted bread. Layer with 1 tablespoon of almond butter, 1 tablespoon of chia seeds, half of a sliced apple, and 1 teaspoon of raw honey.

WEEKS 2, 3, AND 4: Lessen the amount of honey you use each week. Aim for none by week four.

LUNCH: Hummus wrap

HOW TO MAKE IT: Use a sprouted wrap and layer it with organic hummus, lettuce, tomato, and sliced cucumber (or whatever veggies you prefer). Wrap and enjoy!

WEEK 2: Add ⅓ sliced avocado.

WEEK 3: Sprinkle 1 tablespoon of sesame seeds into the wrap.

WEEK 4: Use butter lettuce in place of the sprouted wrap.

AFTERNOON SNACK: Power Bar

HOW TO MAKE IT: See recipe on page 168. Or buy one, but choose a bar that has organic ingredients, with at least 7 grams of protein and less than 10 grams of sugar.

WEEKS 2, 3, AND 4: Experiment with different kinds of bars to see which brand makes you feel best.

DINNER: Large salad with roasted butternut squash and garbanzo beans

HOW TO MAKE IT: Toss together lettuce, broccoli, tomatoes, avocado, carrots, celery, or any other veggie you enjoy. In a pan or oven, slice and roast butternut squash and rinsed garbanzo beans until they are tender. Combine the ingredients for a salad and toss with olive oil and balsamic vinegar.

WEEK 2: Swap lettuce with arugula.

WEEK 3: Swap arugula with kale.

WEEK 4: Return to week one recipe and swap butternut squash with sweet potato.

WEEK 1, DAY 4

BREAKFAST: Nondairy Pancakes

HOW TO MAKE IT: See recipe on page 167.

> **WEEK 2:** Swap out the blueberries with blackberries or strawberries.
>
> **WEEK 3:** Omit the nut butter.
>
> **WEEK 4:** Progressing from week three, swap honey with maple syrup.

LUNCH: Soup and salad

HOW TO MAKE IT: You can get a soup and salad when you're out, but make sure to stay away from creamy dressings, cheese, fried meat, or bacon. Avoid creamy soups and instead opt for broth-based soups. If you are making soup at home, simply roast some veggies, such as sweet potato, cauliflower, or acorn squash, and blend them with coconut milk and spices. Make a big salad and you're done!

> **WEEKS 2, 3, AND 4:** Always opt for low-sodium soups. Each week, decrease soup size and increase salad size. Instead of pouring dressing on the salad, dip your fork into the dressing with each bite.

AFTERNOON SNACK: Power Bar

HOW TO MAKE IT: See recipe on page 168.

> **WEEK 2:** Add 1 teaspoon of chlorella.
>
> **WEEK 3:** Progressing from week two, swap out the hemp seeds with sesame seeds.
>
> **WEEK 4:** Progressing from week three, omit the nut butter.

DINNER: Pasta with meat sauce

HOW TO MAKE IT: Cook pasta according to directions. Sauté ½ cup lean ground turkey, bison, or crumbled tempeh. Add your protein to the sauce, throw in a handful of mushrooms and spinach, and combine with the cooked pasta.

WEEKS 2, 3, AND 4: Lessen pasta and meat portions each week.

WEEK 1, DAY 5

BREAKFAST: Overnight Oats

HOW TO MAKE IT: See recipe on page 166. Make one swap each week as suggested below.

WEEK 2: Swap goji berries with pomegranate seeds.

WEEK 3: Swap chia seeds for ground flaxseeds.

WEEK 4: Swap cacao powder for acai powder.

LUNCH: Burger and sweet potato fries

HOW TO MAKE IT: If you're out, opt for a veggie, bison, or turkey burger whenever possible. Skip the bun and order sweet potato fries or a salad. If you are making your own burger, purchase bison, turkey, or frozen veggie patties. Cook your patties and set aside. Slice up one sweet potato. Toss it with olive oil, pumpkin seeds, and spices, and bake it at 375°F for 30 minutes.

WEEK 2: If you start with a beef burger, swap with bison.

WEEK 3: Swap bison for a turkey burger.

WEEK 4: Swap a turkey burger for a non-soy veggie burger (or make your own using beans, oats, spices, and a chia egg made from 2 tablespoons of chia seeds and 3 tablespoons water.)

AFTERNOON SNACK: Ants on a Log

HOW TO MAKE IT: See recipe on page 179.

> **WEEKS 2, 3, AND 4:** Same!

DINNER: Stir-fry

HOW TO MAKE IT: Cook ½ cup of brown rice and sauté broccoli, Swiss chard, red pepper, and mushrooms with organic tofu. Drizzle with Bragg's Liquid Aminos or coconut aminos (a great substitute for soy sauce).

> **WEEK 2:** Swap brown rice with quinoa. Add one veggie.
>
> **WEEK 3:** Swap quinoa with millet. Add one veggie.
>
> **WEEK 4:** Swap millet with amaranth. Swap tofu with a bean.

WEEK 1, DAY 6

BREAKFAST: Power Greens Shake

HOW TO MAKE IT: See recipe on page 172.

> **WEEK 2:** Add ¼ cup of hemp seeds or hemp protein.
>
> **WEEK 3:** Progressing from week two, add 1 teaspoon chlorella.
>
> **WEEK 4:** Progressing from week three, omit the berries.

LUNCH: Salad with chicken

HOW TO MAKE IT: Toss roasted chicken over a bed of lettuce with some snap peas, celery, roasted acorn squash (optional), a handful of walnuts, and some raisins.

> **WEEKS 2, 3, AND 4:** Swap out your protein each week with fish, garbanzo beans, adzuki beans, black beans, or hemp seeds.

AFTERNOON SNACK: Trail mix

HOW TO MAKE IT: Choose two different nuts (such as walnuts and Brazil nuts) and toss a handful with chia seeds, flaxseeds, or sesame seeds and dried fruit, such as raisins, apricots, figs, or dates.

> **WEEKS 2, 3, AND 4:** Vary the ingredients!

DINNER: Pizza

HOW TO MAKE IT: Purchase an organic crust (or use sprouted tortillas) and top with tomato paste or marinara, fresh organic veggies, and crumbled tempeh. Sprinkle with feta or Daiya nondairy cheese. Bake at 350°F for 12–15 minutes, or until "cheese" has melted. If you're ordering in or eating out, ask that they go light on the cheese and double up on the veggies. Stick to eating two or three pieces and accompany with a small salad.

> **WEEK 2:** Go cheeseless with your pizza, using marinara and veggies instead.
>
> **WEEK 3:** Progressing from week two, opt for a gluten-free crust.
>
> **WEEK 4:** Progressing from week three, stick to just two pieces and pair with a salad.

WEEK 1, DAY 7

BREAKFAST: Detox Green Juice

HOW TO MAKE IT: Grab an organic green juice at a local market or juice bar, or see recipe on page 171.

> **WEEKS 2, 3, AND 4:** Same!

LUNCH: Sandwich

HOW TO MAKE IT: If you're eating out, skip the deli meats and opt for a veggie option instead. At home, make a sandwich with two pieces of sprouted wheat bread, a thin layer of hummus, tofu, lettuce, tomato, and mustard. Serve with veggies or pita chips.

> **WEEKS 2, 3, AND 4:** If you're eating chips, try switching with veggies.

AFTERNOON SNACK: Power Bar

HOW TO MAKE IT: See recipe on page 168.

> **WEEKS 2, 3, AND 4:** Same!

DINNER: Veggie burger

HOW TO MAKE IT: Combine 1 cup of garbanzo beans or black beans with ½ cup of oats, one chia egg composed of 2 tablespoons of chia seeds and 3 tablespoons of water, mustard, and preferred spices in a food processor. Process until sticky. Roll into patties and bake for 20 minutes at 400°F or sauté in grapeseed oil. If you're eating out, order a veggie burger without the bun and opt for a side salad or steamed veggies.

> **WEEK 2:** If making at home, choose a different bean.

> **WEEK 3:** Add sesame, flaxseeds, or hemp seeds into recipe.

> **WEEK 4:** Progressing from week 3, steam the veggies instead of sautéing them.

As you progress, if you find that you are doing well, feel free to make even more tweaks by looking at the Intermediate (page 138) and Advanced (page 145) programs ahead.

Craving Alert!

Got a craving? If you're faced with something you just can't resist, see an ad on TV, or smell something delicious but off-limits, sit with it. Sniff deeper. Imagine indulging in that food from the first bite to the last. Go through the entire experience in your head. Our senses are vastly vivid. If I think back to any food I ate in childhood, I have the ability to still taste that food, just by imagining it in my mind's eye.

So do that. Indulge in your mind. And then think about what happens once the last bite is taken. How will you feel? Where will this get you? Is there something just a little bit healthier that you can "budget" in that will satisfy your craving without blowing your entire day?

Verbalize what you want and why you want it. And then think about how many times you've had that food and what exactly it's done for you.

If you can name three nutritional benefits that that food has, then eat it. If you can think of even one reason why it's *not* beneficial, avoid it. Just make it a rule. You no longer eat that food.

When you are in a relationship and you see someone attractive, do you pursue him or her? Just as you wouldn't cheat on a significant other as impulsively as you would succumb to the drive-through, stop and think about what you're craving, why you're craving it, the pros and cons of giving in, and the realization that you *have* power over food. It has no power over you.

Repeat that to yourself anytime you are faced with temptation.

Intermediate Detox

Thirty-one days of healthier eating should cleanse your system, improve nutrient absorption, and increase fertility odds. During this time you want to focus on foods you can eat in their most natural state. When we eat natural foods that don't have to be cooked, we get live nutrition.

Cooking kills your food, which can put carcinogens into your body, as well as kill vital nutrients in your food. (However, eating gently cooked foods can be beneficial for some people who have more delicate digestive systems and can't necessarily digest all raw food.) For this cleanse, you are going to think about simple foods, allowing your digestive system to work the way it was meant to.

Because you generally have a healthy attitude about food, limiting cooked food to just one meal per day should be easier than you think.

Use these ten basic guidelines as a checklist to visit before meals. Which tips can you use for what meals? Think simply, and you will be on your way to your best body (and mind) yet.

1. **SOAK AND SPROUT YOUR NUTS AND SEEDS.** Contrary to popular belief, eating a handful of nuts or seeds doesn't mean you're getting the proper nutrients they provide. Most nuts and seeds are made to be soaked and sprouted to release all those yummy nutrients. Without water, they are dormant. Water "wakes" them up and makes them easier to absorb and digest. Many people who have nut allergies or have a hard time digesting nuts and seeds don't have an issue if they have been soaked. Because nuts and seeds are essentially asleep, soaking them brings them back to life and promotes a healthy gut, rather than causing bloating and gas. This is an easy swap for everyday life. Tossing water over your nuts or seeds

at night will ensure they are ready to be rinsed and eaten in the morning.

2. START THE DAY WITH A SMOOTHIE PLUS AVOCADO. Consume good fats and sugars early in the day to jump-start metabolism. Fruit is best consumed on an empty stomach, and the morning is a great time to digest these simple sugars. Fruit sugars provide good energy without the crash (unlike caffeine). Popping an avocado (which is a fruit!) into a smoothie provides healthy fats that keep hunger at bay. The fiber aids digestion as well. Experiment with different fruits or greens to see what keeps your energy stoked and your belly full.

3. INCREASE NON-MEAT PROTEIN CONSUMPTION. Increase non-meat proteins by adding quinoa, garbanzo beans, and beans to your meals. Many forms of plant-based proteins in the range of grains, legumes, nuts, and seeds make endless varieties available. Chances are if you eat meat, you stick to the common few: chicken, turkey, and beef. Animal proteins (other than eggs, which are the easiest of animal-based proteins to digest) can take up to forty-eight hours to digest, causing inflammation and a fight-or-flight response in the body. Beans and legumes soaked in filtered water with sea vegetables like kombu or wakame digest quickly and don't cause gas. Try swapping meat proteins with plant-based proteins once or twice a day. The best part? Many plant-based proteins can be eaten raw and simply tossed on a salad or in a smoothie!

4. MAKE YOUR OWN "JUNK" FOODS OR DESSERTS. While you're trying to eliminate desserts from your life, sometimes that ugly sugar devil rears its ugly head. If you're a social butterfly, don't shy away from events because you're afraid you're going to cheat. Go out with friends, have a good time, but save dessert for home. Making an easy avocado pudding or banana ice cream can save you loads of calories and keep your digestive system happy. If you're craving something sweet and have a dehydrator, dehydrate fruits or other foods, such sweet potatoes, to make chips that you can keep with you as easy, sweet snacks. Limit your desserts to once or twice a week to give the body a break.

5. SAY GOOD-BYE TO CHEESE. Who doesn't love a great cheese? Unfortunately, cheese and dairy are full of bacteria or are processed to the point where pharmaceutical-grade drugs have to be included. Eliminating dairy most days of the week will ease inflammation, improve digestion, and prompt weight loss without trying. It will help with bloating as well. And, contrary to popular belief, you aren't going to suffer from a lack of calcium. Amaranth, almonds, apricots, chia seeds, collard greens, dried fruit, quinoa, sea veggies, soy, and sesame seeds are just some of the foods that contain significant amounts of calcium.

6. ADD GREENS TO EVERY MEAL. While you might think adding greens to every meal is impossible, think again. Adding greens at every meal helps alkalize the body, fill you up while keeping calories down, and provide useable energy for a couple of hours. The fiber from the greens will also fill you up and help promote elimination. Start the day with a green smoothie, choose veggies and hummus for a snack, have a huge salad for lunch and some veggies at dinner. Dose your body with minerals and easy-to-digest nutrients.

7. DRINK LESS ALCOHOL. You might eat well, but if the end of your day is capped with a glass of red wine, it's time to revisit your habits. Take a break from your beloved vino or cocktail and see what this does to your waistline and sleep patterns. Cutting out the wine pre-pregnancy will help with the transition as you get closer to conception. Not ready to give it up completely? Limit yourself to one drink two times per week, and always drink a glass of water for every alcoholic beverage you consume.

8. EAT HIGHER-QUALITY PRODUCTS AND PRODUCE. Not eating organic but eating loads of veggies? You may be eating tons of cancer-causing pesticides as well. Make sure to eat the cleanest local veggies possible. Not only do they taste better, they are better for you and will provide a more nutrient-packed punch. Can't afford organic? Go to your local farmers' market and chat with farmers about their practices. Many don't use pesticides but can't label themselves as certified organic because of the high costs involved.

9. START USING APPLE CIDER VINEGAR. Not only can apple cider vinegar clean your house, relieve sunburns, cure yeast infections, improve digestion, and slash serious health risks, it's a natural antibacterial as well. Apple cider can also help lessen joint pain and heartburn, clear up skin problems, and promote circulatory health. It breaks down fats and helps your body use them instead of storing them. Add a tablespoon of apple cider vinegar to your morning smoothie to combat digestive problems and inflammation. When ingested or rubbed on the skin, apple cider vinegar is also an amazing alkalizing agent.

10. ADD FERMENTED FOODS TO YOUR DIET. Fermentation is a metabolic process that converts sugars to acids, gases, or alcohol. Fermentation is a bit of a science if you're doing it yourself, but these foods are incredibly beneficial for your gut. Learn to ferment your own foods, or enjoy a kombucha beverage, sauerkraut, or kimchi. Since fermented foods heal the digestive system and eliminate inflammation from the body, aim to eat these foods at the end of the day.

Ten-Day Omission Period

Which trigger foods do you eat the most often and when? Are they related to stress, convenience, or budgetary restrictions? During your ten-day omission period, target the meals where you eat these foods the most often and swap them with a healthier choice. If caffeine is your crutch, for instance, start your morning with half-caf then switch to black tea, transitioning from there to green tea, herbal tea, and finally, a caffeine-free life. Your goal over these ten days is to omit or switch your crutch foods to ready you for the cleanse.

Three-Week Meal Plan

Because you have a good handle on healthy food, we're going to use a paint-by-numbers approach to your meal plan. Choose a column per meal to mix and match your daily menu. For breakfast, for example, the first column consists of ingredients to make a smoothie, the second for an oatmeal or porridge, and the third to make a power bar. These are just base suggestions, allowing for variety and demonstrating what you can pair together to make quick, easy meals with what you have at home.

Sample meals are below, as well, in case you need some inspiration. Remember, these are just suggestions and ideas. This cleanse has flexibility, which is key. The idea is to keep your meals simple and flavorful using whole foods and fresh herbs. Two days per week, eat one meal of your choice, whether that's at home or at a restaurant.

We are going to stick to eating three meals a day to give the digestive system a chance to rest. Choose which meal you want cooked, and try to keep the rest raw. I typically find it easy to make a giant smoothie in the morning, a raw soup or salad for lunch, and then a cooked dinner at night. If you find that three meals per day doesn't support your physical activity, opt for two snacks during the day. There will be a snack column you can pull from as well. All portions should heed the following:

- Veggies/Greens: Unlimited
- Fruit: One piece is considered one serving or ½ cup
- Grain: One serving is ½ cup cooked. If you are extremely active, you can bump this up to 1 cup cooked.

- Seeds: 2 tablespoons
- Nut butter/Hummus/Spreads: 1–2 tablespoons
- Toppers/Dressings: 1–2 tablespoons
- Protein/Legumes: ½ cup to one cup cooked
- Fermented foods: ½ cup or one kombucha beverage per day

Breakfast: Pick one column

Option 1	Option 2	Option 3
Four greens	One raw grain	One dried fruit
Two fruits	One seed	Two seeds
One seed	One dried fruit	One nut
Two superfoods	One cup nondairy milk	One superfood
One cup nondairy milk	Two toppers	

Lunch: Pick one column

Option 1	Option 2	Option 3
Three leafy greens (such as spinach, collards, or kale)	One sprouted grain	Wrap (lettuce)
One red veggie	One sprouted legume	Hummus or spread
One orange veggie	Two veggies	Two veggies
One seed		
One sprouted legume		
One herb		
Apple cider vinegar and lemon .		
1 tablespoon oil (hemp, olive, coconut, flax, etc.)		

Afternoon Snack: Pick one column

Option 1	Option 2	Option 3
Two dried fruits	One veggie	Two fruits
One seed	One nut butter/ spread	Nondairy milk
One nut	One seed	One seed

Dinner: Pick one column

Option 1	Option 2	Option 3
One protein	One grain	Three veggies
Two veggies	Three veggies	One protein
One topper	One topper	One topper

Meal Ideas

Breakfast	Lunch	Dinner	Snack
Power Greens Shake (page 172)	One pound salad	Stir-fry	Trail mix
Power Bar (page 168)	Raw quinoa bowl	Salad and pasta	Ants on a Log (page 179)
Green Juice (page 186)	Raw soup	Soup and salad	Superfood Veg Smoothie (page 172)
Overnight Oats (page 166)	Quesadilla (page 173)	Raw Pad Thai (page 178)	Power Bar (page 168)
Granola	Avocado Pesto Zoodle Bowl (page 179)	Big burrito	Raw Sprouted Hummus (page 181)
Raw Vegan Oatmeal (page 169)	Sushi rolls	Sushi rolls	Raw Chia Pudding (page 170)
Acai Smoothie (page 171)			

Toppers

- Nutritional yeast
- Raw honey
- Tahini
- Kimchi

Advanced Detox

Though you might not think you need any help in the dietary department, checking in to make sure you're eating enough calories and a wide variety of foods is important while cleansing and prepping for baby.

While you may have eaten raw in the past (or you might eat raw 80 percent of the time), for your plan, you are going 100 percent raw. That's right: all in, baby. By eating 100 percent raw, you will allow the digestive system to break down, utilize, and eliminate all foods. Your goal will be to increase energy, reduce waste, and eradicate all toxins from your system in a short period of time. During your plan, you can focus on those foods that have been proven to boost fertility and use these general guidelines to get you started on your path to a healthy detox!

1. **DRINK GINGER TEA EVERY MORNING.** Ginger helps fight inflammation (and nausea). Fighting inflammation first thing in the morning helps prepare the body for the day. You can grate your own fresh organic ginger into a pot with filtered water and sip before breakfast.

2. **DRINK ALKALINE WATER.** If you think all water is equal, think again. Most bottled water is really just tap water, as there are no strict rules or guidelines as to what's filtered and what's not. Toxins run rampant in our drinking water. If you can, purchase a home alkaline water machine, or buy water from a vendor. Test your blood pH before setting the water pH level. The best way to help heal the body is by making it neutral. A level from 6.5–7.5 is preferable. Not interested in alkaline water? Spring water is your next best bet.

3. **ENJOY JUICING.** If your body functions well and you are healthy, you can throw in a mini juice cleanse for just one day per week or every few weeks. This quick reset is all that is

needed to boost metabolism or eliminate digestive issues. See juice recipes on page 186.

4. EAT MORE. Unless you are a plant-based nutrition expert, you might not be eating *enough*, which can slow down the metabolism and your system. This could be the reason why you're tired (if it's not poor sleep, dehydration, or stress). When eating a high fruit and vegetable diet, you need to eat enough calories to sustain your daily activities. Though your lunch salad may be embarrassingly large, it only amounts to approximately 500 calories or less. When you eat raw, you need to eat a bit more to sustain your activity (unless you are sedentary for most of the day). While it's not vital to count calories, especially if you are eating raw, you want to make sure you are getting proper fuel throughout the day, especially if you are an active woman or training for a sport. (And yes, you can still build muscle being raw.)

5. MAKE YOUR OWN FLOURS. If you are gluten-free and often purchase prepackaged almond (or other) flours to bake your goodies, stop. All packaged goods (even the "good" ones) go through a pasteurization or stabilization process, so they will last longer on a shelf. Real almond flour has to be refrigerated and only lasts about two weeks. Making your own flours by grinding oats or almonds is a great, fresh way to up your nutrient density and cut back on harmful processes.

6. BUY SOME KITCHEN GADGETS. If you love that store-bought organic juice, you know how expensive healthy eating can be. Nix the $9 juice and make one at home instead. Figure out what healthy treats you eat the most, then do some research on what kitchen item might improve your lifestyle. A high-powered blender? A juicer? A dehydrator? A food processor? A spiralizer? A mandolin? If you have a birthday coming up, send a hint to loved ones that these make great gifts as well.

7. EAT FOR YOUR AILMENTS. Chances are you might suffer from some type of ailment from time to time. For example, if you suffer from an autoimmune disorder (there are over 200), nightshade vegetables and fruits, even tomatoes, are not your friend. Nightshades can include banana and jalapeno peppers, cayenne, chile peppers, eggplant, potatoes, goji berries, tomatoes, etc. Learn what veggies/fruits are better for your body, depending on what issues you are suffering from.

8. MAKE YOUR OWN NONDAIRY MILKS. If you already do this, you might try switching up what type of milk you make. If almond milk is your go-to, blend some hemp seeds, soaked cashews, or pumpkin seeds with water and try something new. Choose a different nut or seed every week, add vanilla or dates, and enjoy the variety.

9. NIX THE SUPPLEMENTS. If you are someone who gets giddy when you walk into a health food store (guilty as charged), you might be overdoing it on the supplements. Challenging yourself to get everything you need from food should be your first priority. Supplements are just a backup. If you are eating the way you should, you don't need supplements and vitamins. Your body doesn't recognize pills and powders the same way it recognizes food, so save the money and eat your vitamins instead.

10. PAY ATTENTION TO EXTERNAL HEALTH. We tend to focus on what goes into our bodies, but what goes on *outside* the body is just as important. From the cookware we use and the plastics in our homes to the fire retardants built into our furniture, toxins are everywhere. Your skin is your largest organ. If you want to purchase natural products for your skin, skip the high-priced, multi-list products and raid your kitchen instead. Coconut oil, almond oil, and olive oil make great moisturizers and will not make you greasy! Mix a little sugar with honey and lemon or lime juice for an easy scrub. Use that activated charcoal or spirulina for some inventive eyeliner and your oats for a gentle scrub, or take a bath in it to relieve eczema. Want to "cleanse" your home? Throw away the cleaning products and sprays and use essential oils and vinegar instead. See Chapter Eleven: Detox Your Life for specific tricks and tips!

Complete Proteins

What are complete proteins? The term refers to amino acids, which are the building blocks of protein. There are 20 different amino acids that can form a protein, and nine that the body can't produce on its own. These are called essential amino acids—we need to eat them because we can't make them ourselves. In order to be considered "complete," a protein must contain all nine of these essential amino acids.

While some plant foods can be low in the essential aminos, others are abundant. But, you can get everything you need if you eat a varied diet. For instance, when you combine grains, legumes, nuts, seeds, and veggies (as you would in most meals), these foods become complementary and provide all the essential aminos.

So what plant-based foods or combinations contain all the essential amino acids?

- Amaranth
- Aphanizomenon flos-aquae (algae)
- Buckwheat
- Chia seeds
- Chlorella
- Hemp
- Hummus and pita
- Mycoprotein (Quorn)
- Peanut butter sandwich
- Quinoa
- Rice and beans
- Seitan (contains wheat)
- Soy
- Spirulina with grains or nuts
- Sprouted bread (contains wheat)

Keep this handy list in mind when pairing your meals or when you feel you need an extra dose of protein.

Seven-Day Omission Period

Use this week to take stock of any foods you want to get rid of. Whether it's eggs, meat, caffeine, or that small bit of dairy you indulge in now and then, start phasing these foods out for a full seven days.

Two-Week Meal Plan

Because you just need two weeks, it's imperative to stick to the plan as closely as possible. The more diligent you are to keeping it clean, the easier it will be to detox and prep yourself for pregnancy.

For this cleanse, stick to eating four times per day (three meals and one snack), using a new superfood each day to pop into your diet. Remember, eat when you're hungry and at different times every day. People mindlessly eat every three hours because that's what they think they should do. This cleanse is about tuning in to your body, eating when you're hungry, and refraining when you're not hungry. It's not about a set of rules.

Focus on eating 100 percent raw to promote the easiest digestion, elimination, and absorption of minerals.

Don't be afraid to double your portions of smoothies, salads, burritos, or raw burgers if you feel you need to. Listen to your body and make sure you are adequately hydrated to push all that fiber through the system.

You'll notice that grains are not included in this plan. Feel free to add sprouted grains wherever you see fit (or if you feel like you need something extra). Below is a sample week with tips to get the most success from your cleanse. Make enough to feed one to two people. The juices and smoothies should be around twenty to thirty-two ounces.

Recipes for each main meal can be found starting on page 165. Enjoy!

MORNING BEVERAGE: Ginger Lemon Tea (page 195)

Meal Ideas (Choose One from Each Column)

Breakfast	Lunch	Dinner	Snack
Detox Green Juice (page 171)	Salad (rotate greens daily/ weekly: kale, romaine, spinach, arugula, radicchio, butter lettuce, etc.)	Soup	Superfood Veg Smoothie (page 172)
Superfood Veg Smoothie (page 172)		Sea veggie "noodle" salad	Raw bar
Raw Vegan "Oatmeal" (page 169) with Raw Almond Yogurt (page 170)	Raw Vegan Pad Thai (page 178)	Avocado Pesto Zoodle Bowl (page 179)	Raw yogurt
	Raw burrito	Raw burrito	Raw Chia Pudding (page 170)
	Sandwich wrapped in lettuce or collard greens	Sushi rolls	
	Sushi rolls, minus the rice		

Daily Tips

1. **ROTATE SMOOTHIE SUPERFOOD POWDERS.** Choose between acai berry, chlorella, maca, kelp, and spirulina to take your smoothie up a notch.

2. **ROTATE YOUR OILS.** Choose between grapeseed, flaxseed, olive, coconut, hemp, or avocado oils for salad dressings and sauces.

3. **ROTATE YOUR SEEDS.** Make sure you rotate seeds as much as possible. Choose between flax, chia, hemp, sesame, pumpkin, moringa, and SaviSeeds.

4. **EAT YOUR SEA VEGGIES.** Use sea veggies in your salads, soups, or smoothies. Purchase powders or flakes to toss into smoothies if you don't like the taste.

The Detox While You Are Expecting Athlete

You've probably seen those rare breeds of women who still compete or do CrossFit while pregnant. How do you really know what's safe and what isn't?

Pregnancy is not a time to start a brand-new fitness routine. If your body is used to a particular type of training, you can keep to the same training patterns—just pay attention to how you're feeling during all activities.

Here are some important detox rules for the athletic woman:

Take a look at the ingredients of your favorite protein powders. If they have more than just a few ingredients, nix them. Stick to those that are just one or two ingredients, like hemp protein, brown rice protein, or pea protein.

Stick to sprouts or seeds to get all your protein needs post-workout.

Make sure you are eating enough to sustain your activity level. Figuring out how many calories you burn during your sport is a great starting point.

Make healthy replenishers with coconut water, lemon, and a dash of sea salt to stay hydrated and keep those electrolytes in check.

---

5. EAT YOUR FERMENTED VEGGIES. Kimchi and kraut should be your new best friends. Ferment your own in about three days, or throw a heaping spoon of kimchi on your salad.

6. EAT GARLIC. Use garlic in your dressings; opt for black garlic if available.

7. ROTATE YOUR PROTEINS. Make sure you're getting sprouted beans or legumes a few times per week. Soak and sprout for better absorption (and to keep your diet completely raw). Choose from adzuki, garbanzo beans, lentils, black beans, etc.

8. EAT SPROUTS. Load up on sprouts whenever you can, or make your own.

9. DRINK TEA. At night, see what calming teas you can drink to help flush the system and relax the organs for a good night's sleep.

10. VARY YOUR PROTEIN POWDERS. If you like making smoothies with protein, vary your powders. Choose between pea, hemp, brown rice, cranberry, artichoke, or alfalfa, or try a blend of a few to see what makes you feel best.

CHAPTER ELEVEN

Detox Your Life

From beauty supplies to cleaning products and even contact lens solution, many of the products we use as women are toxic, especially while pregnant or nursing. Because we slap on makeup for most of our lives, we're already at a greater disadvantage than men. We don't ever look at men and think, "God, he needs some foundation," so why do we do it to ourselves? When did we stop going into the world barefaced?

Toxins we apply daily absorb into the skin and affect our health just as much as what we eat and drink. A fast rule: If you can't eat it, don't put it on your skin. Yes, this seems a hard rule to live by, but it's also incredible to see how much better you feel when you nix the junk and start going a bit more natural.

Your Best Face Forward

When I became pregnant, I was on a mission to swap out all of my "semi-natural" products for truly natural products, and this took a lot of research and some help from one of my favorite books, *No More Dirty Looks: The Truth About Your*

Beauty Products—and the Ultimate Guide to Safe and Clean Cosmetics by Siobhan O'Connor and Alexandra Spunt.

After reading this book (which exposes all those hard-to-pronounce words in our beauty products and what they *really* mean), I went around my home and gathered all my standard "go-to" products in terms of cosmetics, soaps, and detergents. I was horrified by what I read.

From paraben-laced shaving cream to an ingredient list a mile long in the Dove beauty bar I once loved to the Moroccan oil shampoo and conditioner I thought was super nontoxic to my beloved Burberry perfume (don't get me started) and even all of my husband's cosmetics, we realized we were indeed toxifying our bodies with everything we used.

On a mission, I wrote down all the recommendations from the book and went to the only place nearby that sold some of these more natural products: Whole Foods Market. While you can get many of these items online, I wanted to at least look at them. I wanted to compare them against other brands. I wanted to smell them and ask questions if I needed to. I wanted to spend some time reading the labels and really get to know what I was putting in and on my body on a daily basis. (Fact: This is good to do *now* with children's products before you're even pregnant, rather than when your child comes down with eczema or that awful mystery rash and you are struggling to figure out what the hell to buy.)

As I gathered new products, I tried to refrain from getting too excited. I'd been down this road before with certain products and come home to have my beautiful new face wash break me out after just one use. And natural deodorants? Pardon my French, but most of them can go f*** themselves. Instead of finding a natural deodorant that actually worked, I simply stopped using them. And with a clean diet and healthy lifestyle, I realized I didn't even *need* to wear deodorant. To be free of body odor and not rely on something to mask it? It is completely possible.

(It's important to note that in recent research by Keele University, aluminum from standard deodorant was found in breast tissue. While the jury has always been out on whether aluminum and parabens contribute to breast cancer, do yourself a favor: Stop using regular deodorant. If you read the ingredient list, this alone should give you pause. Why would you put all of those harsh chemicals that close to breast tissue?)

As I continued my search, I realized what I really wanted was food-grade, quality items for my skin. When I thought of what I might have already exposed Sophie to in utero, I became furious and a bit fearful. But, I was also hopeful that I could bring her into a world that was cleaner than my world, and one that she would continue to perpetuate (if she wanted to).

So, loading up on some natural purchases (which, yes, are more expensive than their cheaper counterparts), I began to make some comparisons. While there are a ton of natural finds out there, here are some of my favorites. When choosing body washes or lotions, always opt for the ultra-sensitive brand, as these are the most stripped of harsh ingredients and fragrances.

Recommended Brands

SHAMPOO AND CONDITIONER: John Masters Organics, Giovanni, California Baby, Everyday Coconut, Goldies Natural Beauty, Aubrey, Dr. Hauschka, CTonics, Alaffia

At-home option: Use coconut oil as a conditioner, or after conditioning, use a small amount of argan oil in hair. Make your own shampoo with baking soda, lemon, and apple cider vinegar, or skip the shampooing altogether and jump on the cowashing bandwagon, which skips shampooing and instead uses conditioner as the star player.

DEODORANT: Natural Grooming (for men), Lady Anti-Smellum, Lavanila, Weleda, Tom's

At-home option: Mix baking soda with melted coconut oil, essential oils, and arrowroot powder.

BODY WASH: California Baby, SheaMoisture, Pangea Organics, Dr. Bronner's, Jurlique

SHAVING CREAM: I opt for conditioner or body wash as shaving cream. I also use natural shampoo to wash off my makeup brushes.

TOOTHPASTE: Jason Powersmile, Nature's Gate, Tom's, Neem

At-home option: Mix baking soda, water, sea salt, and peppermint essential oil.

MOISTURIZER (BODY): SheaMoisture, Egyptian Magic, vitamin E oil

At-home option: Mix argan oil with your favorite lotion for an extra dose of moisture.

MOISTURIZER (FACE): Acure, Juice Beauty, Jurlique, John Masters Organics, Evan Healy, Dr. Andrew Weil for Origins, Ren

At-home option: Mix argan oil with a little coconut oil (if you're not acne prone) or use aloe or jojoba oil.

FACE WASH: Acure, Andalou Naturals, Juice Beauty, Jurlique, Whole Foods Market Triple-Milled Organic Soap, Ren, Even Healy, Patyka

At-home option: Combine sugar, oats, honey, lemon or lime juice, and baking soda.

BLEMISH TREATMENT: Acure, Juice Beauty, Jurlique, Organic Apoteke, Burt's Bees, Jason, Alba Botanica, Yes To, Avalon Organics, Weleda, Lavera

At-home option: Tea tree oil, apple cider vinegar, Wisdom of Ages Advantage Liquid Concentrate (referred to as ALC and composed of grapefruit seed extract, jasmine tea, and green tea), witch hazel

MAKEUP: Mineral Fusion, ZuZu, Dr. Hauschka, Physicians Formula, Alba Royal Jelly (for lips), EcoTools (for brushes), Lavera, Nvey Eco, RMS Beauty, Jane Iredale, Laura Mercier, Bare Escentuals, Alima Pure, Josie Maran, W3LL People, 100% Pure

At-home option: Make your own eyeliner or eye shadow from activated charcoal and spirulina powder; make your own lip or cheek stains with a little piece of beet. See what you have laying around the house that can be used to give a little touch of color.

PERFUME: Make your own blend from essential oils and a good base, like vanilla or almond extract.

SUNSCREEN: Caribbean Solutions, Kiss My Face, California Baby, Aubrey Organics, Soléo, Lavera

TAMPONS: Nix the toxic cotton and other materials and opt for a DivaCup instead.

Time to Clean House

Go to your cleaning products right now and throw them all away. I can't tell you how thankful I was that I got rid of any harsh chemicals, especially once I had a crawling baby on my hands. If she breaks into the cabinet and gets a hold of the vinegar and water bottle we use to clean our home? No biggie. If she gets a bottle of bleach? It could kill her.

From fancy sprays to harsh chemicals in our laundry detergent, there are other options out there. You just have to know where to look. Read the entire ingredient list on your all-purpose cleaners. Here are some pre-screened recommendations (remember to always get fragrance free):

CLEANING PRODUCTS, INCLUDING DISHWASHING LIQUID AND DETERGENT: Seventh Generation, Mrs. Meyer's, Method, Common Good, Bon Ami.

At-home options: Mix a spray bottle with ¾ cup water, ¼ cup white distilled vinegar, and lemon juice or lemon essential oil. Use for all surfaces. Baking soda, lemon juice, and salt make a great natural scrub. Use ALC drops mixed with water to spray fruits and vegetables or to clean surfaces.

LAUNDRY DETERGENT: Seventh Generation, Soap Nuts, Mrs. Meyer's, Ecos, 365 Everyday Value, Ecover Zero

The Blacklist

So, what are the truly "bad news" ingredients to stay away from when looking at ingredient lists? Thanks to the authors of *No More Dirty Looks*, the extensive alphabetical list below is always handy for inspecting your cosmetics and cleaners. If you look at this list, you'll notice most of the bad ingredients end in -ate, -ete, -ide, -en, -ene, -oate, and -ol, and are generally just hard to pronounce. Always research ingredients you are uncertain about and familiarize yourself with this list for all future products.

- 1, 4-Benzene (and variations like Benzenediamine, Benzenediol, etc.)
- 1, 4-Dioxane
- Aluminum (including variations with chloride, hydrochloride, chlorohydrate, hydroxybromide, oxide, zirconium, etc.)
- Ammonium lauryl sulfate
- Ammonium persulfate
- Benzalkonium chloride

- Boric acid (and several variations beginning with bor)
- Bronopol, aka 2-bromo-2-nitropropane-1,3-diol
- Butylated hydroxyanisole (BHA)
- Butylated hydroxytoluene
- Butylparaben
- Ceteareth (including all number variations)
- Chloroacetamide
- Coal tar
- Cocamide dea
- Cocamide mea
- D&C red 30 lake
- D&C violet 2
- Dea oleth-3 phosphate
- Dea-cetyl phosphate
- Diazolidinyl urea
- Dibutyl phthalate
- Diethanolamine (DEA)
- Dihydroxoybenzene
- Disodium EDTA
- Dmdm hydantoin
- Ethylparaben
- Eugenol
- FD&C dyes
- Ficus carica or fig extract
- Formaldehyde (including when followed by resin, solution, etc.)
- Formalin
- Formic aldehyde
- Fragrance
- Homosalate
- Hydroquinone
- Hydroxybenzoate
- Hydroxybenzoic acid
- Hydroxyphenol
- Imidazolidinyl urea
- Iodopropynl butylcarbamate
- Isobutylparaben
- Lauramide DEA
- Lanolin
- Laureth-7
- Lead acetate
- Lecithin
- Light liquid paraffin
- Manganese sulfate
- Methly aldehyde
- Methylbenzene
- Methylparaben
- Mineral oil
- Monoethanolamine (MEA)
- Myristamide DEA
- Nonoxynol
- Octinoxate
- Octoxynol (usually followed by a number)
- Ocytl-methoxycinnamate
- Oleamide DEA
- Oxybenzone
- Paba
- Padimate-o
- Paraffin
- Parfum

- Peg (followed by any number)
- Perfume
- Petrolatum
- Petroleum distillatte
- Phenol
- Phenoxyethanol
- Placental extract
- Polyethylene
- Polyethylene glycol
- Polyethylene terephyhalate
- Polyoxyethylene
- Polysorbate-80
- Potassium persulfate
- P-phennylenediamine
- Propyl acetate
- Propylene glycol
- Propylparaben
- Quaternium-15
- Resorcinol
- Saccharin
- Sodium laureth sulfate
- Sodium lauryl sulfate
- Sodium metabisulfate
- Sodium methylparaben
- Stearamide mea
- Sotddard solvent
- Talc
- Talcum poser
- Teflon
- Tea lauryl sulfate
- Tretrasodium edta
- Thimerosal
- Thioglycolic acid
- Toluene
- Triclosan
- Triethanolamine
- Triphenolphosphate

A Makeup Intervention

I recently chatted with Ashlee Piper, editor-in-chief of *The Little Foxes* (www.thelilfoxes.com) to find out the do's and don'ts when shifting to a more natural cosmetic life.

What are the big no-nos in terms of ingredients we should stay away from in our makeup, cosmetics, and cleaning products?

Ashlee: I personally avoid animal ingredients and harsh chemicals like bleach, formaldehyde, acids, silicones, parabens, sulfates, non-natural preservatives, artificial colors (which can get very tricky with color cosmetics), and plastic microbeads (horrible for skin and the environment). After using natural products for years, synthetic fragrances give me serious headaches and breakouts, so I avoid those as well. In addition to ingredients I avoid, I never buy anything that isn't explicitly cruelty-free, meaning that the product has not been tested on animals during any phase of production, formulation, or ingredient sourcing. I don't think you can ever be beautiful if you're harming animals in the process.

What are the best natural makeup brands out there?

Ashlee: I am really loving 100% Pure, which makes gorgeous fruit-pigmented color cosmetics like lipsticks and blushes. I also adore Pacifica and Josie Maran (not 100% natural, but very gentle and formulated to be caring to skin and the environment). I also have a host of skincare companies I adore: Aster & Bay; La Bella Figura Beauty; Vapour Organic Beauty; One Love Organics; Flo + Theo; Desert Essence; Pelle Beauty; May Lindstrom Skin; Lina Hanson; Earth Tu Face; Shea Terra; R.L. Linden and Co; Mullein and Sparrow; Gressa Skin; and many others. I am a facial oil junkie—give me a vial of a moisturizing oil blend, and I am a happy girl. For fragrance, I love LUSH, Kuumba Made, Aroma M Perfumes, and Pacifica, to name a few. For hair, I am really loving Rahua, Natu, and Maijan—all are vegan, cruelty-free, and easy on the toxins. For personal care, I adore North Coast Organics natural deodorant cream and Eco-Dent whitening toothpaste powder. I am also obsessed with konjac sponges, which are derived from vegetable fiber. They are so marvelous for removing makeup (in concert with an oil cleanser), very gently exfoliating, and are so gentle you can wash newborns with them. When you're done with the sponge, you can put it in the bottom of a potted plant to help distribute hydration. Genius!

Do you have any at-home recipes for making your own face wash, perfume, body wash, toothpaste, or deodorant?

Ashlee: I use cornstarch, a little baking soda, and a few drops of essential oils (whatever I'm feeling that day) sifted into a shaker container to make a wonderful dry shampoo for light hair. I love this super-simple recipe because I can bring this with me when I travel, and it doubles as a cooling and refreshing body powder to keep you dry when the weather gets sticky. For perfume, I often use essential oils to freshen clothes, my skin, and to shake into my laundry, or the carpet before I vacuum; I also sprinkle it in my running shoes or suitcase. I make my own facial serums and oil cleansers. I use a base oil of jojoba for normal skin, or almond or avocado for dry, winter skin. Then I blend in other, more bespoke oils and ingredients like macadamia, olive, marula, rose hip, sea buckthorn, raspberry leaf, sesame oils, green tea, rosewater, vegetable glycerine, coconut water, neroli, and essential oils (sandalwood, lavender, jasmine, geranium, lemongrass, mint, etc.) to make serums or oil cleansers (my favorite way to remove makeup!) that feel right for whatever my skin is needing at the moment. This requires a little upfront expense of buying the oils in bulk, but you save so much money in the long run and you get incredible value for your money—and everything is tailored to you!

For home care, I make my own spray surface cleaner using vinegar (the smell fades after a while), purified water, fresh muddled basil, and cedar and sage oils (which are antibacterial). I put it all in a charming, old-school glass spray bottle and it smells like heaven. Added bonus: Cedarwood oil naturally deters pests like bedbugs, ticks, fleas, roaches, and ants, so I spray this mixture on my pups as a natural flea deterrent and my home is pest-free naturally. For surfaces that require scrubbing, nothing, and I mean nothing, works better than baking soda and lemon essential oil. It shines up metal like a dream, cleans tile and grout, and gets grime off of damn near anything. People think you have to bleach the heck out of everything and use antibacterial soap and hand sanitizer at every turn, but what they don't realize is that those things are not only toxic, but they compromise your immune system. Germs are a natural part of life, and it's healthy to be exposed to a normal amount—that's how our body adapts and strengthens its immune response. Constantly bombarding our bodies and environments with chemicals, antibiotics, and antibacterial elements weakens our body's responses and actually makes us less healthy. Cleaning with natural products ensures a clean home without the chemical shit storm.

How important do you think it is to pay just as much attention to what we put on our bodies as to what we put in our bodies?

Ashlee: Incredibly important! I see some of the fittest, most health-conscious clean eaters slather themselves with conventional products that are literally the equivalent of drinking a vat of mystery fast-food fryer oil. Your body is a symbiotic system. As with food, if your body does not recognize something, it cannot process or use it and will store it as a toxin, which can often lead to a systemic buildup or allergic reaction. I think it's incredibly important to ensure your personal care products, home care products, and products you're using for your little ones are as clean and kind as possible, because your skin is your largest organ. It takes and breathes in everything on it and around it.

Can natural makeup really work as well as "regular" makeup?

Ashlee: Absolutely. In fact, in many cases, I think natural makeup works better. For instance, all skin needs hydration, but chemicalized skincare "wisdom" tells us that we need chemicals like acids and peroxides to dry out acne or harsh microbeads and scrubbing brushes to exfoliate. Much natural makeup and skincare is built on a foundation of hydration, synergy, and gentleness, and I think this is important as we age or live in different climates and conditions. I love how hydrating natural foundations are, and in most cases, I think natural makeup is like good skincare with dewy color. And who doesn't like that?

The Skinny

As you can see, there's a whole fun world of cosmetics and natural products that work better and are safer for the environment (and for you and your impending baby). Making your own cleaners or beauty products is fun, inexpensive, and can often work better than most of the harsh chemicals and expensive brands on the market.

This was one of the most enjoyable parts of my ongoing detox. Start digging and making swaps to see how much better you can look, how much cleaner your house can get, and how much better you will feel from keeping those toxins at bay.

CHAPTER TWELVE

DBYE Recipes

On the following pages, you will find some easy, nutrient-dense recipes that take less than twenty minutes to prepare. Jazz them up any way you want to. I've left the palate basic so you can start easy then play around with ingredients as you see fit. There are also swap suggestions for some of the recipes to get as much variety as possible.

Even if you hate to cook, don't think of these recipes as "cooking." They are not labor-intensive. Most are raw and take just a few minutes to throw together. While most of us love eating out, the truth is that we can't control the quality of ingredients we consume or the amount of salt, sugar, or oil that's being put into our food by restaurants. By eating in even three nights a week, you will change your health for the better.

Please note that all recipes are plant-based and most will make *at least* two big servings or three or four smaller servings. As you come off your cleanse, experiment by adding in your own chosen ingredients or swapping with ingredients you feel more comfortable with.

Enjoy!

OVERNIGHT OATS

Switch the oats with different grains or pseudograins, such as millet, quinoa, or buckwheat to keep this dish interesting. *Makes 2 servings*

½ cup oats

¼ cup raisins

¼ cup chia seeds

1 teaspoon ground cinnamon

1 teaspoon cacao powder (optional)

Nondairy milk, to cover

1 tablespoon dried goji berries (optional)

Drizzle of raw honey (optional)

1. In a resealable glass bowl, pour in the oats, raisins, chia seeds, cinnamon, and cacao powder, if using. Add enough nondairy milk to cover the oats well. Stir and place a lid on the bowl. Pop in the refrigerator for a few hours or overnight.

2. In the morning, drizzle with goji berries and raw honey, if using.

NONDAIRY PANCAKES

Feel free to use different add-ins, such as pure pumpkin, berries, or seeds. *Makes 9 pancakes*

2 tablespoons chia seeds

½ banana, mashed

1 tablespoon vanilla extract

1 tablespoon apple cider vinegar

1 cup nondairy milk (soy milk recommended)

⅔ cup oats or oat flour

½ teaspoon baking soda

1 teaspoon baking powder

1 teaspoon ground cinnamon

1 tablespoon hemp seeds (optional)

2 tablespoons chopped walnuts (optional)

⅓ cup blueberries (optional)

1 teaspoon grated ginger (optional)

1 tablespoon grapeseed or unrefined, virgin coconut oil, for cooking (optional)

Sliced banana, for topping (optional)

⅓ cup nondairy chocolate chips, for topping (optional)

Honey or molasses, for topping

1. In a liquid-measuring cup, dump chia seeds, mashed banana, vanilla, and apple cider vinegar. Pour nondairy milk on top (it will probably reach the 1½-cup mark with the add-ins). Stir and let sit until chia seeds plump, approximately 5 minutes.

2. In a Magic Bullet or blender, grind your oats to a flour. Dump ground oats in a medium bowl with baking soda, baking powder, cinnamon, and hemp seeds, if using, and stir lightly.

3. Pour the wet mixture into the bowl with your dry ingredients. Mix until well combined. If the mixture is too thick, pour in more nondairy milk.

4. Stir in the walnuts, blueberries, and ginger, if using.

5. Heat a griddle over medium heat. Spread 1 tablespoon of coconut oil or grapeseed oil (or forgo oil altogether) on the griddle. Once the griddle is hot, use a dry measuring cup to ladle batter onto it ¼ cup at a time. Cook 2–3 minutes per side, until golden brown.

6. Top with sliced banana and chocolate chips, if using, and a little honey or molasses.

POWER BAR

To change things up, experiment with different nut or seed butters, nuts, and seeds for a variety of flavors. *Makes 20–30 balls*

10 dates, pitted

⅓ cup hemp seeds

⅓ cup almonds

⅓ cup sunflower butter

⅓ cup chia seeds

⅓ cup oats

2 tablespoons cacao powder

1 teaspoon spirulina powder

1 tablespoon dark chocolate chips (optional)

Juice of 1–2 lemons

1. In a food processor, process dates until they are chopped up. Add in all of the other ingredients, except lemon juice.

2. Process until the mixture starts to combine, then trickle in the lemon juice until the mixture starts to clump into a ball. Make sure the mixture isn't too wet. (If it's too dry, add more lemon juice. If it's too wet, sprinkle in more oats.)

3. Dump the mixture onto parchment paper. Pinch off sections and roll them into balls. Pop in fridge or freezer for 10 minutes then enjoy.

RAW VEGAN "OATMEAL"

This recipe was adapted from Jess Rice Andrews, chef de cuisine at Avo in Nashville, Tennessee, and creator of the blog *My Poor Tired Liver*.   *Makes 4 servings*

5 organic red or green apples, cored and washed

2 tablespoons lemon juice

1 cup coarsely chopped walnuts, divided

1 cup pitted Medjool dates

1 teaspoon ground cinnamon

½ cup raw pumpkin seeds

½ cup hemp seeds

⅓ cup sunflower seeds

1 cup raisins

Chopped fresh fruit (optional)

1. In a food processor, process 2 of the apples with the lemon juice, ½ cup of walnuts, and the pitted dates until they reach the consistency of applesauce.

2. Dice the remaining 3 apples into bite-size pieces and combine with the applesauce.

3. Add all of the remaining ingredients and stir.

4. Garnish with fresh fruit, if using, additional cinnamon, or local, raw honey.

RAW ALMOND YOGURT

This recipe was adapted from Jennifer Weems, creator of Raw Food Effect. Tip on peeling the almonds: Simply pinch the almond between your thumb and index finger after soaking and the skins will pop off. *Makes 4 servings*

1 cup almonds, soaked overnight and peeled

Juice of ½ lemon

Agave or raw honey, to taste

1 teaspoon almond or vanilla extract, to taste

¾ cup water, or as needed

3–4 probiotic capsules, opened

1. Add almonds, lemon juice, sweetener, and extract to a blender with ½ cup of water. Keep blending and adding water until the desired consistency is reached.

2. Add the powder from the probiotic capsules and blend again.

3. Store your yogurt in the refrigerator and consume within two to three days.

RAW CHIA PUDDING

This recipe was adapted from Jess Rice Andrews, chef de cuisine at Avo in Nashville, Tennessee, and creator of the blog *My Poor Tired Liver*. *Makes 2 servings*

2 tablespoons raw chia seeds

1 cup homemade almond milk (page 187)

⅔ cup chopped fresh berries, divided

½ teaspoon ground cardamom

⅓ cup soaked nuts

⅓ cup pomegranate seeds

⅓ cup hemp seeds

1. Stir chia seeds into the almond milk. Add ⅓ cup of chopped berries and cardamom and stir.

2. Allow pudding to set in your fridge for 2 hours or overnight.

3. Top with the rest of the berries, soaked nuts, and pomegranate and hemp seeds.

ACAI SMOOTHIE

Makes 2 servings

1 pack pure acai puree

½ cup frozen strawberries

1 frozen banana

1 tablespoon hemp seeds

1 tablespoon flaxseeds

1 teaspoon cacao nibs

Nondairy milk or water, to blend

Coconut flakes, for topping (optional)

Raw granola, for topping (optional)

Blend first seven ingredients until thick. Top with coconut flakes and raw granola, if using.

GREEN DREAM SHAKE

Makes 2 servings

1 frozen banana

⅓ cup frozen strawberries

⅓ cup spinach

⅓ cup de-stemmed kale

⅓ cup romaine lettuce

⅓ cup parsley

Juice of 1 lemon

⅓ cup hemp seeds

1 teaspoon chlorella powder

½ teaspoon moringa powder

1–1½ cups nondairy milk or coconut water

Blend all ingredients until smooth. Add more nondairy milk or coconut water if consistency is too thick.

DETOX GREEN JUICE

Makes 2 servings

1 head romaine lettuce

1 bunch de-stemmed kale

1 bunch spinach

½ bunch parsley

4 Granny Smith apples

1 bunch celery

1 lemon

1 piece ginger

Juice all ingredients and serve immediately. If you don't have a juicer, blend all ingredients and strain through a nut milk bag or cheesecloth.

SUPERFOOD FRUIT SMOOTHIE

Makes 2 servings

2 kiwis

1 green apple

1 acai berry frozen pouch

3 ounces frozen or fresh blueberries

3 ounces frozen or fresh strawberries

3 ounces frozen sweet tart cherries

1 tablespoon maca powder

1 banana

2 cups nondairy milk (adjust according to how thick or thin you like smoothies)

Blend all ingredients and consume immediately.

SUPERFOOD VEG SMOOTHIE

If this is too "veg" for you, add one frozen banana to the mix. *Makes 2 servings*

1 avocado, chopped and frozen

⅓ cup de-stemmed kale

⅓ cup romaine lettuce

⅓ cup spinach

⅓ cup parsley

⅓ cup cilantro

Juice of 1 lime

½ teaspoon moringa powder

1 teaspoon chlorella powder

½ teaspoon spirulina powder

½ teaspoon kelp flakes

Blend and consume immediately.

POWER GREENS SHAKE

Makes 2 servings

1 frozen banana

½ cup frozen berries

⅓ cup kale

⅓ cup romaine lettuce

⅓ cup spinach

Pinch of cilantro

Juice of 1 lemon

1 cup nondairy milk

Blend and consume immediately.

CHOCOLATE ALMOND BUTTER SHAKE

Makes 2 servings

1 frozen banana

½ cup frozen strawberries

1 tablespoon cacao powder

1 cup almond milk

1 tablespoon almond butter

¼ cup flaxseeds

Pinch of ground cinnamon

Blend and consume immediately.

QUESADILLA

For a hint of sweetness, add a cooked sweet potato. In place of store-bought Daiya, you can also make your own homemade nut cheese by blending soaked nuts, garlic, lemon juice, and nutritional yeast. *Makes 2 servings*

2 sprouted tortillas

4 tablespoons hummus

Sprinkle of mozzarella Daiya or homemade nut cheese

⅓ cup spinach

Dash of oregano

Sprinkle of cilantro

Unrefined, virgin coconut or grapeseed oil, for cooking (optional)

1. Layer tortillas with hummus, mozzarella Daiya, spinach, oregano, and cilantro. Fold and eat cold.

2. To eat warm, heat coconut or grapeseed oil in a skillet over medium heat. Cook layered tortilla 2–3 minutes per side. Slice and enjoy.

CREAMY ASPARAGUS SOUP

This tasty recipe was adapted from Heather Crosby, author of *YumUniverse* and founder of YumUniverse.com. The soup is equally delicious served chilled. *Makes 2 servings*

1 bunch asparagus (about 25–30 stalks)

1 tablespoon unrefined, virgin coconut oil

1 yellow onion, diced

1 teaspoon fresh thyme, roughly chopped

4 cups pure water

2 teaspoons fresh lime juice

½ teaspoon sea salt (add more to taste)

¼ cup cashews, soaked for 4 hours (or sunflower seeds)

Fresh, cracked pepper, to taste

1. Wash the asparagus and slice it into tiny disks.

2. In a large stockpot, heat coconut oil and onion over medium-high heat for 7 minutes. Stir occasionally.

3. Add asparagus and cook together for 2–3 minutes.

4. Add thyme leaves to the stockpot and stir.

5. Add the water to stockpot and bring to a boil.

6. Reduce heat and simmer for 5 minutes. Remove from heat.

7. Transfer soup to blender. Add lime juice, salt, and cashews and puree until ultra-smooth.

8. Serve hot with fresh, cracked pepper.

BIG BURRITO

Makes 4 servings

Grapeseed oil, for cooking

1 package crumbled tempeh, sautéed

Ground cumin, to taste

Ground turmeric, to taste

Pinch of cayenne

2 cloves garlic, minced

½ cup beans, mashed or refried

4 sprouted wraps, collard greens, or lettuce leaves

1–2 tablespoons hummus (optional)

1 teaspoon tahini

1 avocado, mashed, mixed with juice of ½ lemon

⅓ cup slaw

SLAW

¼ whole red cabbage, chopped

½ bunch kale, de-stemmed and finely chopped

2 carrots, finely julienned

Juice of 1 lemon

Drizzle of olive oil

Pinch of sea salt

1. Make the slaw by stirring all of the ingredients together until well combined. Set aside.

2. In a sauté pan, heat the grapeseed oil over medium heat. Crumble the tempeh with the back of a fork. Toss in pan with cumin, turmeric, cayenne, and garlic and cook until "done," approximately 5 minutes.

3. In a separate pan, add the refried or mashed beans. Heat until warm.

4. Once done, heat your wrap or lay out your collard greens or lettuce leaves, ribs removed. Layer hummus, tahini, avocado, beans, tempeh, and slaw. Wrap and enjoy.

JICAMA SALAD AND DRESSING

Adapted from Reboot Health and Wellness. *Makes 2 servings*

2 cups finely diced jicama

½ cup finely diced celery

½ cup finely diced red onion

¼ avocado, mashed

Parsley, for garnish

SALAD DRESSING

2 tablespoons tahini

¼ teaspoon ground cumin

1 ½ tablespoons lemon juice

2 tablespoons water

2 tablespoons fresh dill or parsley

¼ teaspoon tamari

¼ teaspoon raw honey or agave

Sea salt, to taste

Pinch of white pepper

Pinch of chili powder or paprika

1. In a bowl, combine all of the salad ingredients, except parsley, and set aside.

2. To make the dressing, blend all of the ingredients in a blender until smooth (should be thick) and mix into jicama mixture. Garnish with parsley and serve.

TOMATO AND BEET PISTACHIO SALAD

Makes 2 servings

1 beet, spiralized

3 medium tomatoes, sliced into thin rounds

2 tablespoons olive or grapeseed oil

2 tablespoons rice wine vinegar or balsamic vinegar

1½ teaspoons grated fresh ginger

½ teaspoon raw honey

Pinch of sea salt

⅓ cup shelled pistachios, chopped

1. In a bowl toss spiralized beets with tomatoes.

2. In a separate bowl, mix the rest of the ingredients (minus the pistachios) and whisk until smooth. This will be your dressing.

3. Massage your dressing into the beet noodles and tomatoes. Toss in pistachios and serve.

AVOCADO CARROT GINGER SUSHI ROLLS

Makes 12 rolls

⅓ cup sprouted brown rice

2 nori sheets

½ avocado, peeled and cut into strips

1 carrot, cut into thin sticks

1 small thumb ginger, peeled and minced

½ cucumber, cut into sticks

SAUCE (OPTIONAL)

Splash of apple cider vinegar

1 teaspoon organic stone-ground mustard

1 small piece peeled ginger

1-2 tablespoons water, for consistency

1. Cook the brown rice according to the package directions. Allow to cool slightly.

2. Spread out both nori sheets side by side with their shiny sides down on the cutting board (make sure to read the instructions to see if they need any pre-treatment before eating). Scoop the rice in an even layer over the entirety of each nori sheet and layer the rest of the ingredients on top.

3. Using a sushi roller (or just doing it yourself), tightly roll the nori sheets from one end to the other. You may need to lightly wet the loose end with water to get it to stick when wrapping. You can keep the wraps whole or cut them into rolls using a very sharp knife.

4. To make the sauce, blend all of the ingredients until smooth.

5. Present your sushi rolls alongside a serving of dipping sauce, if using.

RAW VEGAN PAD THAI

This recipe was adapted from Jess Rice Andrews, chef de cuisine at Avo in Nashville, Tennessee, and creator of the blog *My Poor Tired Liver*. *Makes 4 servings*

PASTA

2 whole carrots, peeled with potato peeler to create noodles

1 large zucchini, spiralized

1 daikon radish, spiralized

1 red bell pepper, thinly sliced into strips

⅓ cup fresh basil, chopped

⅓ cup fresh parsley, chopped

Juice of 1 lime

Cracked red pepper or fresh jalapenos, to taste

SAUCE

1 cup raw almond butter

1 thumb chopped and peeled fresh ginger

⅓ cup water

¼ cup lemon juice

¼ cup agave or real maple syrup

3 cloves garlic

1 small jalapeno pepper (most of the seeds removed)

GARNISH

Fresh cilantro, chopped

½ cup cashews (or soaked almonds), coarsely chopped

Lime wedges

1. Toss all of the pasta ingredients together in a large bowl until well mixed.

2. Blend all of the sauce ingredients in a high-speed blender and pour over the noodles.

3. Serve with cilantro and cashews on top and a wedge of fresh lime.

AVOCADO PESTO ZOODLE BOWL

This recipe was adapted from Jess Rice Andrews, chef de cuisine at Avo in Nashville, Tennessee, and creator of the blog *My Poor Tired Liver*.   *Makes 2 servings*

1 large zucchini, peeled with potato peeler or spiralized to create noodles	Pinch of sea salt

RAW PESTO

3 cups raw spinach	⅓ cup water
½ cup fresh basil	⅓ cup lemon juice
½ avocado	1 teaspoon apple cider vinegar
1 clove garlic, crushed and allowed to sit for 10 minutes	Sea salt and pepper, to taste

1. Sprinkle sea salt over your zucchini noodles to break them down a little so they are soft and noodlelike before serving. Set aside.

2. Add all of the pesto ingredients to a food processor and pulse until well-combined and mostly smooth. It should be thick like a paste.

3. Spoon pesto into your bowl of zucchini noodles and toss until they are coated.

ANTS ON A LOG

Makes 4 logs

2 celery stalks	Raisins
Nut butter such as almond, sunflower, or cashew	Sesame seeds

Slice the celery stalks in half. Spread them with the nut butter. Drop raisins and sesame seeds on the butter.

BASIC CARROT FLAX CRACKERS

Adapted from the Reboot Health and Wellness website (www
.reboothealthandwellness). *Makes 30 crackers*

2 cups fresh carrot juice

2 cups fresh carrot pulp

2 cups golden flaxseeds, pre-soaked
for 8 hours into a nice gel

1 teaspoon white pepper

1½ teaspoons sea salt

1. Use a blender, nut milk bag, or juicer to make your carrot
   juice and pulp.

2. Combine all ingredients in a bowl. Mix thoroughly with
   hands or use an electric mixer.

3. Using an offset spatula, spread 1½ cups of mixture onto a
   dehydrator tray outfitted with a teflex sheet.

4. Dehydrate for 8 hours and flip onto a dehydrator tray
   outfitted with just the screen. Dehydrate until the crackers
   reach the desired level of crispiness (typically another 8–12
   hours).

RAW SPROUTED HUMMUS

If you don't have dried garbanzo beans you can use canned, but the recipe won't be considered "raw." *Makes 4 servings*

1 cup dried garbanzo beans	Juice of 2 lemons
2 tablespoons tahini	¼ cup water
1–2 tablespoons olive oil for blending, plus more for garnish	Sea salt, to taste
	Paprika, to garnish (optional)
1–2 large garlic gloves	

1. Place the dry beans in a large bowl and cover them with purified water. Let them sit for 8–12 hours. Rinse and drain. Leave the beans in the bowl until tails begin to sprout (around 2 days). Rinse and drain the beans every 10 hours during this process. If you want to skip the soaking and sprouting process, use canned garbanzos instead.

2. Once tails are sprouted, place all of the ingredients (except paprika) in blender or food processor and blend until creamy. Add more water if needed. Sprinkle with paprika (if using) and a drizzle of olive oil and serve.

TAHINI SAUCE/DRESSING

Makes 2 servings

2 tablespoons tahini

1 tablespoon mustard

1-2 tablespoons water

1 teaspoon horseradish (optional)

Whisk all ingredients together with a fork until smooth. Too thick? Add more water.

RAW VEGAN RANCH DRESSING

This recipe was adapted from Jess Rice Andrews, chef de cuisine at Avo in Nashville, Tennessee, and creator of the blog *My Poor Tired Liver*. *Makes 4 servings*

¼ cup fresh, chopped dill

2 cups raw cashews (soaked for at least 2 hours)

¼ cup sauerkraut juice

1 teaspoon sea salt

2 garlic cloves

3 tablespoons nutritional yeast

1 tablespoon raw apple cider vinegar

Spring water, for blending

1. Setting fresh dill aside, combine all other ingredients in a high-speed blender and process until smooth.

2. Add water as needed until dressing reaches desired consistency.

3. Stir in fresh dill and serve.

EASY BROWNIES

Adapted from the Reboot Health and Wellness website (www.reboothealthandwellness). *Makes 10 brownies*

2 cups walnuts, soaked and dehydrated

5 tablespoons pitted Medjool dates

6 tablespoons cacao powder

1 teaspoon vanilla or chocolate extract

¼ cup dried fruit, such as raisins, cherries, or apricots

¼ cup water

1. Place walnuts in a food processor fitted with an S-blade and process until they reach the consistency of meal.

2. Loosely separate the dates and add them to the food processor. Process with the walnuts until they are well combined. Add the cacao powder and extract and process again.

3. Add the dried fruit and sprinkle a few drops of water (about 1 tablespoon) and pulse a few times just to mix. Continue adding water until you reach the ¼ cup or desired consistency. Do not overprocess.

4. Pack the mixture firmly into a 7×7-inch brownie pan. Chill for 2 hours, slice, and serve. You can also refrigerate for 1 week stored in an airtight container.

RAW VEGAN CHOCOLATE DIP

This recipe was adapted from Jess Rice Andrews, chef de cuisine at Avo in Nashville, Tennessee, and creator of the blog *My Poor Tired Liver*. *Makes 4 servings*

1 cup raw cacao or carob powder

1 cup pitted Medjool dates

1-inch piece vanilla bean

1 teaspoon ground cinnamon

½ cup coconut water, to blend

Combine all ingredients in a high-speed blender and blend until smooth. Adjust the amount of coconut water to achieve desired consistency.

A DIY Juice Cleanse

As previously mentioned in the book, juice cleanses are not for everyone. Usually reserved for those dealing with serious illnesses, juicing should always be approached carefully and with thought.

However, if you clean up your diet and want to try one day of juicing before or after this program, this is one extra step you can take to cleanse the system and reboot it for health. This is *not* necessary to maintain optimal health, but it can offer many health benefits. Because store-bought cleanses can be expensive, you can make a cleanse yourself for a fraction of the cost.

For the following one-day juice cleanse, you will enjoy five juices and one homemade nut milk throughout the day. If you are extending this to a two- or three-day cleanse, be sure to make your juices the day you consume them.

GREEN JUICE

This should be the first and third juice you drink each day. *Makes 1 serving*

5 celery stalks

1 large green apple

1 cup de-stemmed kale

1 cucumber

3 romaine leaves

⅓ cup spinach

1 small lemon

Juice all ingredients and enjoy.

PINEAPPLE APPLE MINT

Consume this juice second. *Makes 1 serving*

⅓ pineapple

1 large green apple

⅓ cup mint

Juice all ingredients and enjoy.

SPICY LEMONADE

This should be the fourth juice you consume each day. *Makes 1 serving*

2 lemons

1 tablespoon agave nectar or raw honey

Dash of cayenne pepper

2 cups filtered water

Juice the 2 lemons. Mix agave or raw honey and cayenne into the lemon juice. Pour mixture into a large mason jar and fill it with water. Consume immediately.

CARROT APPLE BEET

This should be the fifth juice you consume each day. *Makes 1 serving*

1 large green apple

2 beets

5 large carrots

1 large thumb ginger

1 small lemon

Juice all ingredients and serve.

NUT MILK

This should be the last "juice" you consume. You can try it using different nuts, such as cashews, Brazil nuts, or even walnuts. *Makes 1 serving*

3 ounces raw almonds, soaked overnight and drained

2 cups filtered water

1 tablespoon raw honey or 1 date, pitted

1 teaspoon ground cinnamon

1 teaspoon vanilla extract

Place all of the ingredients in blender. Blend on high until well-blended, then strain through a nut milk bag or cheesecloth.

CHAPTER THIRTEEN

I'm Pregnant...
Now What?

You're pregnant! Congratulations! Now everything should fall into place, right? Whether you have planned for a baby for years or this is a complete surprise, no one said pregnancy would be easy. For those lucky few, pregnancy is the most enjoyable time in their lives; but others may feel like strangers in their own skin. It can be overwhelming. It can make you feel like an alien in a world of humans, and sometimes it feels like no one understands. (But I do.)

However, there are ways to cope. Eating well, getting plenty of rest, and finding ways not to stress are vital. Trust me—all of the things we worry about (Will my baby be healthy? What kind of baby shower will we have? What car seat do we get? Can I have sex? Do I *want* to have sex? I *don't* want to have sex! Will I *ever* want to have sex?) will pale in comparison once the baby is born.

Trust me: You don't need to read every book, article, or forum. People have been raising babies for centuries without the input of every blogger and expert in the world. (Just watch the documentary *Babies* to show you how spoiled we are in America.) Cease the questions, put down the baby books (except this one, of course), and just *go with the flow*.

Though I had cleansed myself pre-pregnancy, once I became pregnant, the stresses began to pile on. Suddenly, being "fly-by-the-seat-of-our-pants" freelancers felt like the dumbest thing in the entire world. No "real" insurance. No idea about schools or daycare or doctors or hospitals or what the hell we were going to do. I became so stressed, I'm sure I affected Sophie's hormonal pattern. Pregnancy is not a time for stress; it's a time to relax and let life unfold.

Having a partner who makes you laugh (or finding ways to laugh) is just as important as eating healthy. Feeling supported, joyful, and fulfilled should be on that top priority list—just as much as devising that perfect birth plan.

And of course, focusing on things you *can* control.

Eat for Two...but Not Really

So what's something you can control while pregnant? Eating! Contrary to popular belief, we only need about 80 extra calories per day the first trimester (or none if you're at a healthy weight), 250–300 the second, and 400–450 the third. This equates to an apple in the first trimester, one apple and 2 tablespoons of nut butter in the second trimester, or a serving of black beans, quinoa, avocado, and some veggies in the third—that's it.

While this seems negligible, it's not. Our bodies, while pregnant, absorb more nutrients from what we eat. Our bodies become more efficient, therefore the baby takes what it needs (hence, being irrationally tired) and we get the rest.

What does 250–300 extra calories really look like?

- Smoothie made with 1 cup of nondairy milk, 1 banana, and 2 tablespoons of nut butter
- 2 slices of sprouted toast with 1 tablespoon of nut butter and 10 raisins
- 8 ounces of nondairy yogurt mixed with ½ cup of fruit and 1 ounce of granola
- 1 Power Bar (page 168) and 1 piece of fruit
- 1 cup of cooked brown rice and ½ cup beans, cooked
- 1 pita and 4 tablespoons of hummus

What About Vitamins and Minerals?

How important are vitamins and minerals before and during pregnancy? In this day and age, we'll pop a multivitamin and think the bases are covered. However, our bodies know the difference between real food and a synthetic vitamin. And most vitamins on the market have extremely high doses of certain common vitamins that we can easily obtain through food.

Vitamins and minerals, or micronutrients, perform hundreds of vital functions in the body. Considered essential nutrients, they help shore up bones, heal wounds, and bolster the immune system. They also convert food into energy and repair cellular damage.

Think of vitamin supplementation as an insurance policy. It should be low dosage and taken only when necessary. (Omega-3s are often the only caveat to this, as many people do not get the proper dosages of omega-3 in relation to omega-6.) People often pop copious amount of vitamin C, zinc, or vitamin B12 and think they will be able to slash colds, increase energy, or increase the healing process. However, just like the damage response from eating bad foods, high dosages of synthetic vitamins can wreak havoc on our bodies, especially while pregnant.

The best bet is to get your blood work done to see if you have any deficiencies *first* before supplementation begins. Because popping a vitamin is not a parallel return on your investment as you exceed daily requirements, focus on getting all the nutrients you can from actual food, as they are digested better (and it's hard to overdose on vitamins supplied through food).

However, when you are pregnant, it's usually suggested to take a prenatal. But how do you know which ones are best? Opting for vitamins and minerals derived directly from food is *always* preferred. Many brands now source their vitamins directly from whole foods. Always check the labels and read the ingredients (or ask a nutritionist for help) to choose which is best for you.

Joanne Marie writes in "How Does a Poor Diet Affect Fetal Development?" that low vitamin C has been linked to abnormal heart development, while low vitamin A may slow cell division and interfere with lung, liver, and heart development in developing fetuses. Deficiency in vitamin D can slow general growth and development of bones in fetuses, while low intake of vitamin K could interfere with development of the face and teeth and with mineral deposition in fetal bones. Fetuses also need *all* of the B vitamins, but one of these, folate, is especially important. Low folate levels may cause spina bifida, a condition in which development of the fetal spinal cord and vertebral column is abnormal. Minerals such as calcium, iron, zinc, and iodine are also crucial for both the fetus and the mother, helping ensure a normal pregnancy and healthy full-term baby.

While it's important to pay attention to all the macro and micronutrients with any diet, if you are venturing into a plant-based diet while pregnant, it's useful to pay special attention to the following areas of your diet as well:

PROTEIN: An additional 10–15 grams of protein per day should be supplied to the diet. If you are a vegetarian, these can come from sources like hemp, legumes, nuts, and whole grains (other sources include enriched nondairy milk, tofu, tempeh, nut butters, seeds, and higher-protein pseudograins, such as quinoa).

VITAMIN B12: This vitamin is used for tissue synthesis. It is essential for a healthy nervous system and smooth muscle movement. B12 is not always plentiful in plant foods. Good sources include: chlorella, miso, kombucha, nutritional yeast, fortified soymilk and tofu, and fortified, ready-to-eat cereals. Moringa, which is a plant indigenous to African and Asia, supplies over 100 percent of your daily needs in just half a teaspoon! You can purchase it in powder form and sprinkle it in smoothies.

IRON: Many women suffer from anemia, even during pregnancy. Iron is essential for red blood cell health. Enough iron ensures the body is able to deliver oxygen-rich blood to the extremities. Make sure to eat plenty of leafy green veggies, such as spinach or kale, dried beans, and legumes (especially split peas), pumpkin seeds, and dried fruits. If necessary, an iron supplement may be recommended if you can't keep your iron levels up. (However, it's always best to get iron from food as supplements can back you up and be harsh on your system.) Vitamin C helps with the absorption of iron as well.

CALCIUM/VITAMIN D: These vitamins and minerals help bones and teeth, which are important to a child's development. Ninety-five percent of the body's calcium is stored in the skeleton. Vitamin D helps the body absorb calcium. A little exposure to sunlight per day is good for vitamin D, as is fortified nondairy milk. Despite what the billion-dollar dairy industry would like you to believe, you don't have to ingest dairy to get enough calcium (as dairy is incredibly acidic and may actually leach calcium from our bones. Too much salt can do the same thing). Eat plenty of leafy greens like spinach and collards, unhulled sesame seeds, tahini, calcium-fortified tofu, soymilk or hemp milk, broccoli rabe, figs, blackstrap molasses, and sea vegetables. Research calcium and vitamin D supplements to see which are best for you.

ZINC: Necessary for growth and development, zinc allows the body to use dietary protein as building blocks to regenerate muscles. It also helps in proper immune function. You can find this mineral in pseudograins (such as buckwheat, quinoa, wild rice, and amaranth), pumpkin seeds, nutritional yeast, peas, beans, brown rice, spinach, nuts, tofu, and tempeh.

FOLATE: Folate is a B vitamin that is found naturally in foods. In supplement form, it is referred to as folic acid. You can up your intake of folate to around 400 mcg per day even before you become pregnant, and around 600 mcg if you are pregnant. Eating plenty of dark, leafy greens, legumes, pseudograins, whole grains, and nutritional yeast provides plenty of folate.

The good news? If you eat a balanced diet, you can usually meet and sometimes exceed your nutritional needs. Eating a balanced diet rich in whole foods with very little saturated fat, processed foods, and sugar, as well as taking a high-quality prenatal vitamin, will ensure a better pregnancy.

Decide what your diet will consist of when you get pregnant. Where will you get those vitamins and minerals? The DHA? The omegas? The protein? Are going to have a plant-based pregnancy, a raw pregnancy, a regular diet, or a paleo pregnancy? It's important to research all of the proper nutritional needs specific to you—your weight, your health issues, and your baby. Again, if you feel the need to supplement, consult your physician to have the appropriate blood work done to see if you even need supplementation. Remember that you should not focus on *any* supplementation to detox while pregnant, as this can harm you and the fetus.

Pregnancy Recipes

No matter how healthy you are, you can still suffer from nausea or cravings while pregnant. Indulging in healthier fare helps keep your blood sugar stable and avoid unnecessary weight gain. The following recipes helped me with nausea, cravings, and lack of energy when I felt like sleeping (or vomiting) for a year.

GINGER LEMON TEA

Makes 1 serving

1 cup hot water

1 thumb fresh ginger, peeled

Juice of 1 lemon

1. Pour hot water over ginger and fresh-squeezed lemon juice.
2. Let cool. Sip slowly and try not to think of food.
3. Remember that this discomfort will end one day and you will look back fondly to this time, when your vagina was normal and you had no stretch marks and you could sleep whenever you wanted to.
4. Blame your husband.
5. Rest.

RAW GRANOLA

Makes 1 serving

2 cups raw old-fashioned oats

2 tablespoons raisins

2 tablespoons hemp seeds

2 tablespoons raw almond butter

1–2 tablespoons raw agave or honey, to taste

1. Mix all ingredients together in a bowl and spread on a baking sheet or in a glass baking dish.
2. Pop in the refrigerator for an hour. Eat cold.
3. Try to stop yourself at one serving. Realize that this is never going to happen.
4. Keep eating.
5. Finish entire recipe and make another batch.
6. Never tell husband about this recipe so you don't have to share it.
7. Go take a nap from eating so many raisins, but congratulate yourself for providing your baby with hemp and iron from said raisins.

COCOA CHIA PUDDING

Makes 2 servings

1 tablespoon raw cacao nibs

1 date, pitted

1 avocado

2 tablespoons chia seeds

1 banana

1. Blend all ingredients, chill in the refrigerator, and serve.

2. Eat a spoonful and realize how much it resembles baby poop.

3. Realize you will soon become so desensitized to baby poop, you won't even flinch.

4. Realize you will soon become so obsessed with baby poop that you will have numerous pictures on your iPhone of potty poops to remind you what a healthy colon your daughter or son has.

5. Eat the rest of the pudding and vow not to make another. Realize that you have just had the only relaxation you will have for the entire day.

NUTRIENT-BOOST JUICE

Makes 1 serving

2 Granny Smith apples	⅓ cup spinach
6 celery stalks	⅓ cup de-stemmed kale leaves
1 cucumber	1 lime
⅓ cup collard greens	Slice of ginger

1. Juice all ingredients and serve.

2. Pretend it's spiked with alcohol.

3. Mourn the loss of having a glass of wine with dinner or a mojito on vacation for at least the next couple of years (welcome to breast-feeding!).

4. Drink these often before the nausea gets you and you can't stand the sight of a green vegetable without running to the bathroom.

5. Blame your husband for what is happening to you, then offer him a green juice as an apology.

SPROUTED TOAST WITH COCONUT OIL AND ALMOND BUTTER

Makes 1 serving

2 slices sprouted bread

1 teaspoon coconut oil

1 teaspoon almond butter

Drizzle of raw honey

1 teaspoon chia seeds

⅓ cup blueberries

1. Toast the 2 slices of sprouted bread.

2. Slather on coconut oil and almond butter. Drizzle with honey and sprinkle chia seeds and berries on top.

3. Stuff your face with this simple, delectable mixture.

4. Marvel at how much coconut oil tastes like butter (even though you don't like butter).

5. Buy six packages of frozen sprouted bread to hoard for your entire pregnancy (and after).

6. Watch as jars of coconut oil and almond butter disappear at a disturbing pace.

7. Again, blame it on your husband.

RAW HUMMUS WRAP

Makes 1 serving

2 large collard leaves or 1 sheet of nori wrap

2 tablespoons hummus

1 teaspoon hot mustard (optional)

½ zucchini, thinly sliced into strips

½ cup thinly sliced sprouted organic tofu

½ avocado, thinly sliced

1. Cut collards away from thick stem. Lay flat. If using nori, place a nori sheet, shiny side down, on a cutting board.

2. Spoon in hummus and mustard.

3. Layer all other ingredients on top.

4. Roll up, slice, and eat cold.

5. Show your husband your creation. Listen as he makes a joke about a green penis erupting with vegetables.

6. Roll your eyes and tell him he can't have one.

7. Fight over wrap until innards fall onto your lap and you are so hungry you scoop them up and eat them anyway.

8. Watch as your hubby looks at you in disgust.

9. Tell him, "I'm pregnant, you idiot. I'd lick chocolate off the floor if it was available."

10. Listen to him say you can lick chocolate off his balls.

11. Tell him that's how you got into this mess in the first place.

12. Go take a nap.

CHAPTER FOURTEEN

Maintenance for Detoxing Post-Baby

Once you have a baby, it can feel like health is the last thing on your mind. Besides sleep, a maid, a nanny, and a shrink, you probably want a pot of coffee injected directly into your veins. With huge hormonal surges and feelings of being overwhelmed, sore, and exhausted, your post-baby time can feel like the most exhilarating, messy, and uncertain time in your life.

When should you get back into a healthy routine post-baby? The simple answer? When your body feels ready. Remember that it took nine months to make a baby, so give yourself at least nine months to return to a "pre-pregnancy" state before you decide you want to detox or drop a significant amount of weight. While you might not ever have the time to be as painstakingly precise as you were pre-baby, some simple tips and tricks to keeping a healthy, sustainable diet can go a long way when you don't have time to spend hours in the kitchen.

The suggestions below can help aid in your post-baby detox (or any time you are feeling the need to regain optimal health).

MAKE YOUR BREAKFAST GREEN. No matter what you typically eat first thing in the morning, opt for a green juice or green smoothie at least three mornings per week. Want to get really fancy? Start with a green juice and opt for a green smoothie a few hours later. An easy way to get all of your greens, detoxify the system, and boost hydration at the start of the day.

EAT THE COLORS OF THE RAINBOW DAILY. While it might be easy to eat the same sandwich for lunch and pasta for dinner once you have a baby, you and your baby can't subsist on brown foods. Instead, think about eating a plethora of colors throughout the day, or focus on one color per week and try to stick to that hue as the basis for every meal. As kids grow, this is a fun way to have them pick out their fruits and veggies and plan "red" or "purple" meals.

JUICE ONE DAY A MONTH. If you're not nursing (or have enough milk stored in the freezer), juice for one day to jump-start the body, allow the digestive system to rest, and reset the system.

ENJOY A MONTHLY EPSOM SALT BATH. While someone might not twist your arm to take a bath, bathing with Epsom salts can help pull toxins from the body and cleanse your system. If baths aren't your thing, research foot baths, which have also been proven to pull toxins from the system, help with joint inflammation, remove parasites, etc. Research the best salts and level of cleansing for your body.

DO INTERMITTENT FASTING. Choose a few days out of the month, or even one day, and drop your calories by 25 percent (this is not recommended if nursing). This is a great, effortless way to get your body into a short caloric deficit and give the body a great jump-start to cleansing. See Chapter Ten for steps on figuring out your baseline calories.

Your Seven-Day Week

The following rules for each day of the week offer flexibility to go with the flow while maintaining discipline to eat well. Tack this list up where you can see it and just choose one rule to follow each day every day when you are getting back into a healthy routine or decide you are ready to detox postbaby. This allows you to be gentle and forgiving with yourself while still implementing healthy guidelines. These rules also encourage detoxification in a safe way, even if you're nursing. Before you go grocery shopping every week, raid your shelves and refrigerator to see what you have first, so you don't waste money. Reorganize the fridge, salvage perishables if you can, and trash the rest.

START WITH A GREEN SMOOTHIE. Yes, this was also in the daily tips above, but most of us won't start every day green. So at least pick one day a week when you can. Load up that shake with spinach, kale, romaine, parsley and whatever else green you can find. Eat regularly for the rest of the day.

START WITH A GREEN SMOOTHIE AND HAVE A CLEAN SALAD BEFORE LUNCH. Make it a super-healthy day by starting off strong with your smoothie or juice, then having a salad before your regular meal. Eat whatever you want for lunch—just have your greens first (without all the bacon, cheese, or heavy dressings). Eat regularly for dinner.

NO DESSERTS. Though you might not eat desserts daily or even most days, if you had a brownie yesterday, make today the day you skip desserts. This goes for sugary drinks as well as chocolate or even excess fruit. Think of it as a low-sugar day.

NO PROCESSED FOOD. This one is harder than you think. For one day, don't eat anything from a box, bag, can, or package. Nothing that's been altered from its original form.

EAT COMPLETELY RAW. Opt for clean, easy, raw meals the entire day. If this seems tough, start with some overnight raw oats, have a smoothie for lunch, and enjoy a salad for dinner. This can meet all your requirements and give that digestive system a break.

EAT MONO MEALS. What does this mean? This means today, you are not going to combine any foods. You can eat whatever you want, but eat the foods separately. If you want fruit, eat a huge bowl of just one fruit. Want fish for dinner? Have fish. Hungry later? Then down that rice or veggie. This will equal to more of a snacking kind of day, but see how you feel and if it helps your digestive system assimilate and eliminate.

EAT LIGHT TO HEAVY. Start with lighter meals (a juice), head to salads or veggie-based soups, and end with your heavier carbs, like pastas or proteins (and even a dessert).

Post-Pregnancy Exercises

Once you've been cleared to exercise, if you're like me, you want to get back in shape ASAP. I found that my glutes, which used to be high, round, and tight, somehow shifted during pregnancy, and I had to work extra hard to get them into some semblance of their pre-pregnancy shape. (I also blame this on hours and hours of sitting and being in my thirties. Mom butt, be gone!)

Finding some easy exercises you can do for arms, abs, legs, and butt with or without your baby are great ways to stay active and keep your metabolism revved. You can do all of these exercises from the comfort of your home, whenever you feel like it (or at the gym or even in your own backyard). What no one tells you about the beginning of motherhood? There's often *a lot* of sitting and nursing your baby, which can lead to copious amounts of eating and couch time. Combat that with easy five- to ten-minute stints of exercise throughout the day.

CHAPTER FIFTEEN

DBYE Baby Recipes

First things first: Baby food is expensive. Plus, you don't know what factory those fruits and veggies have been through or how long they've been sitting in those jars. Next to breast milk, making your own organic baby food can be the best thing for your little one. But, I know, I know—who has the time? *You do.* With easy gadgets (Magic Bullet or a blender) and a little bit of organization, you can cheaply make all of your baby's meals with minimal effort.

Not only will your baby feel better, you will marvel at the lack of waste and how easy the cleanup is, not to mention all the extra money you will save simply by making your own food. Fruit and veggie packets average about $2 (or more) per packet. If your child eats one every day, that's $14 a week, or $728 per year! Nix the popular trend, buy some of the reusable "green" pouches online and fill them with healthier (and fresher) concoctions. If money isn't incentive enough, we've probably all heard those horror stories of a child going to eat from a packet, only to pull out a worm or something equally gross. By making your own food from whole ingredients, you are serving fresh food. No processing plants. No spoilage. No additives. Fresh from you to them.

The first six months of a child's life is usually easier in the eating department (if you're nursing). If you are nursing, make sure you're getting adequate nutrition, plenty of water, and an extra 500 calories per day, and that you're abstaining from all those yummy things like excess sugar, alcohol, and caffeine.

Once your little one gives you the signals that he or she is ready for solid food, it can be overwhelming to know where to start. There are many different recommendations, most of which suggest starting with rice cereal. Rather than start your child's palate on a grain, consider pureed fruits and veggies. They are easy to digest, much more flavorful, and nutritious. There are many principles one can follow, such as baby-led weaning (where you never puree the food but instead let the child get used to different shapes and textures by eating food in its natural form). My school of thought after a scary choking incident with a piece of apple is that we would stick to purees for a while. She would learn to eat solids eventually (and she did). Research options to see what you're most comfortable with and what works best for your family.

No matter what you start with, remember that what you begin feeding your baby can have a lasting impression. Pureed soups, puddings, and smoothies will become your new best friend. As your child grows, you can begin to weave in some fun superfoods, swap those unhealthy cookies for homemade ones, and help provide the adequate nutrition that is so vital to them as they grow.

All recipes below are safe once children can start eating solid foods. Recipes with seeds or seed butters are best suited for kids whose digestive systems are more developed and who are allowed to start eating seeds. If you're unsure, check with your pediatrician to see when your child can indulge.

HOMEMADE BABY FOOD (6+ MONTHS)

Choose one fruit or veggie from the list below:

Avocado	Plum
Banana	Hachiya persimmon
Mango	Sweet potato, steamed or baked
Peach	Butternut squash, steamed or baked

Mix your fruit or veggie of choice by hand or with a blender with ¼ teaspoon of chlorella and ¼ teaspoon of spirulina powder or kelp flakes. Stir and serve.

HOLY GUACAMOLE (6+ MONTHS)

This guac is easy, tasty, and perfect for dipping veggies or pita chips. The lemon juice helps prevent the guacamole from oxidizing.

1 avocado, mashed with a fork	Juice of ½ lemon

Stir lemon juice and avocado together until chunky.

PUREED CEREALS (10+ MONTHS)

Pick one item from the list below:

Amaranth	Millet
Barley	Oats
Buckwheat	Quinoa

Soak your cereal item overnight. In the morning, rinse, cook, and then puree. You can add a bit of nondairy milk to make it creamier in texture.

SMOOTHIES (10–12+ MONTHS)

From the list below, choose two fruits (if using frozen, use ⅓ cup), one seed (1 tablespoon), one superfood (¼ teaspoon powder), and a nondairy milk (½–1 cup).

Fruits	Seeds	Superfood	Nondairy milk
Banana	Hemp	Chlorella	Almond
Peach	Chia	Wheat grass	Coconut
Cherries	Flax	Spirulina	Hemp
Pear	Sesame	Moringa	Rice
Apple	Pumpkin	Coconut	
Blueberries			
Blackberries			
Mango			
Avocado			

Blend ingredients with ice and rotate choices often.

JUICES (10+ MONTHS)

The various fruits and veggies in this recipe offer a wide variety of flavors.

1–2 carrots

1–2 celery stalks

1 cucumber

1–2 green apples

1 thumb ginger

½ cup kale

½ lemon

A few sprigs mint

⅓ cup parsley

½ cup romaine lettuce

½ cup spinach

Juice (or blend and then strain) all of the fruits and veggies and serve immediately.

PUMPKIN SOUP (10+ MONTHS)

½ cup canned organic pure pumpkin   1 cup coconut milk

1 tablespoon tahini

Blend ingredients on high speed until slightly warmed.

CACAO PUDDING (10+ MONTHS)

½ avocado, frozen   1 teaspoon cacao

1 banana, frozen

Blend and serve immediately.

SWEET SUNFLOWER SOUP (10+ MONTHS)

1 small sweet potato, steamed, with   1 tablespoon sunflower butter
skin removed
                                      1 cup coconut milk

Combine all ingredients and blend on high until slightly warmed.

BUTTERNUT SQUASH SOUP (10+ MONTHS)

1 small butternut squash, peeled and   1 cup almond milk
cubed, steamed or baked
                                       1 teaspoon ground cinnamon

Blend on high until slightly warmed.

POPSICLES (12+ MONTHS)

Grab a Popsicle mold at a local store and have fun with different shapes. You can also inject molds with breast milk while the baby is younger and teething.

COCONUT AND WATERMELON POP

½ cup coconut water   ½ cup watermelon

Blend on high and pour into Popsicle mold. Freeze and serve.

PINEAPPLE MANGO

½ cup diced pineapple   ½ cup coconut water

½ cup diced mango

Blend on high and pour into Popsicle mold. Freeze and serve.

BANANA COCONUT CHIA

½ cup coconut water   1 tablespoon chia seeds

½ cup banana

Blend on high and pour into Popsicle mold. Freeze and serve.

BABY SUSHI (12+ MONTHS)

1 nori sheet

⅓ avocado, mashed

¼ cup grated carrot

2 heaping tablespoons cooked brown rice

1 tablespoon hummus (optional)

1 teaspoon sesame seeds

1. Lay nori sheet flat with the shiny side up.

2. Spoon mashed avocado, grated carrot, brown rice, hummus, and sesame seeds evenly along sheet and gently roll up.

3. Slice into rolls.

PORRIDGE (18+ MONTHS)

½ cup oats, buckwheat groats, quinoa, or millet

1 cup water

TOPPINGS

Nondairy milk, to taste

Berries, to taste

Raisins, to taste

Ground cinnamon, to taste

1. Combine water and your choice of grain or quinoa. Bring to a boil, reduce heat, and cook, covered, until done.

2. Blend the cooked grains or quinoa with nondairy milk, berries, raisins, and cinnamon for a smooth porridge. As they get older, skip the blending and just stir in the toppings.

TODDLER PANCAKES (18+ MONTHS)

I make these for my daughter once a week and she loves them. Once you get comfortable, you don't even have to measure anything out. Just dump in a bowl, mix, and go! *Makes 9 small pancakes*

2 tablespoons chia seeds

½ banana, mashed

1 tablespoon apple cider vinegar

1 cup nondairy milk

½–1 cup oats

1 teaspoon baking powder

½ teaspoon baking soda

1 teaspoon ground cinnamon

1 tablespoon hemp seeds (optional)

⅓ cup blueberries

1 tablespoon grapeseed or coconut oil, for cooking (optional)

⅓ banana, sliced (optional)

⅓ cup nondairy chocolate chips, for topping (optional)

Honey or maple syrup, for topping (optional)

1. In a measuring cup, dump chia seeds, mashed banana, and apple cider vinegar. Pour nondairy milk on top (it will probably reach the 1½ cup mark with the add-ins). Stir and let sit until chia seeds plump, approximately 5 minutes.

2. In a Magic Bullet or blender, grind oats to a flour. Dump in a medium bowl with baking powder, baking soda, cinnamon, and hemp seeds, if using. Stir lightly.

3. Pour wet mixture into dry. Mix until well combined. If mixture is too runny, add in more flour.

4. Stir in blueberries.

5. Heat a griddle over medium heat. Spread coconut oil or grapeseed oil (or forgo oil altogether) on griddle. Once griddle is hot, ladle the pancakes onto the griddle (I use a ¼ cup dry measuring cup). Cook 2–3 minutes per side, until golden brown.

6. Top with sliced banana, chocolate chips, and a little honey or maple syrup, if using.

"FRIED" ALMOND BUTTER/BANANA SANDWICH
(18+ MONTHS)

Kids love peanut butter and jelly. Give them a healthier spin on this old classic. One Degree Organic Veganics and Silver Hills sprouted breads are my personal favorites.

Makes 1 serving

1 tablespoon coconut oil, for frying	½ banana, sliced or smashed
2 slices sprouted bread	1 teaspoon sesame seeds
2 tablespoons raw almond butter	⅓ cup nondairy chocolate chips (optional)

1. Heat coconut oil in a skillet over medium to medium-low heat.

2. Assemble your sandwich by spreading the almond butter on the bread and layering the banana. Sprinkle on sesame seeds and chocolate chips, if desired.

3. Place sandwich in the skillet and cook a few minutes per side, until browned. Slice and serve immediately.

CHOCOLATE ALMOND MILK (18+ MONTHS)

1 cup almonds, soaked overnight for 8–12 hours

3 cups water

1 heaping tablespoon raw cacao powder

3 dates, pitted

1 teaspoon vanilla extract (optional)

1. Dump all ingredients in a blender. Blend on high speed until well combined.

2. Over a large bowl, pour mixture into a nut milk bag or a cheesecloth and let drain. Gently press down and squeeze on bag to extract milk until all mixture is released.

3. Bottle in a mason jar. Milk should be consumed within 3–5 days.

BANANA CHOCOLATE CHIP ICE CREAM

3 frozen bananas

1 frozen avocado (optional)

1 tablespoon nut butter

1 tablespoon dark chocolate chips

Place all ingredients in a blender and blend on high speed, scraping down sides as needed, until creamy. Enjoy!

A Final Word

As you press forward on this journey, know that the answers to any questions you have can be varied. You can find books, articles, gurus, doctors, holistic practitioners, and experts who will tell you many different things. You may have even read a few things in this book that you disagree with or have heard the exact opposite of.

This is what I encourage you to do: *Trust your judgment.* You are an individual, which means nothing out there will be just right for you if it's packaged for the masses. If you are eager to learn, learn as much as you can from as many people as you can, but then apply the pieces of information you want to what works in *your* life. Do what's feasible for you and your family. Do what makes you happy.

As you will soon see (or may already know), when you become a parent, you are bombarded with opinions (solicited or not) about who you should be as a parent and what's best for your child. Don't consult books or friends—learn your own way.

This is your journey, your cleanse, and that special time in your life before you get pregnant and start a family. Take some time to think about what you really want, and remember that flexibility goes a long way. Be open.

Find out how to heal, stay centered, and cleanse, and don't forget to have fun in the process. And once you have that baby, enjoy every exhausting, beautiful moment. It flies by...and it is *all* worth it.

Remember: "The part can never be well unless the whole is well." — Plato

Good luck!

References

American Pregnancy Association. "Preconception Health for Men," last updated on November 11, 2012.
http://americanpregnancy.org/gettingpregnant/menpreconception.htm

Anderson, Cindy. "The Importance of Nutrition in Pregnancy for Lifelong Health," last modified on September 28, 2010.
http://www.ars.usda.gov/News/docs.htm?docid=20977

Animal Liberation Front. "USDA's Official Number of Animals Killed for Food," retrieved on July 15, 2014.
http://www.animalliberationfront.com/Practical/FactoryFarm/USDAnumbers.htm

Baby Centre. "Inside Pregnancy: How Food Reaches Your Baby," retrieved on July 15, 2014.
http://www.babycentre.co.uk/v1049111/inside-pregnancy-how-food-reaches-your-baby

Brown University Health Education. "Alcohol & Your Body," retrieved on July 10, 2014.
http://www.brown.edu/Student_Services/Health_Services/Health_Education/alcohol,_tobacco,_&_other_drugs/alcohol/alcohol_&_your_body.php

Crosby, Heather. "How to Make Kombucha Tea," retrieved on July 8, 2014.
http://yumuniverse.com/how-to-make-kombucha-tea/

Detoxed News. "A Glance at the History of Detoxification," retrieved on July 15, 2014.
http://blog.thedetoxmarket.com/glow-1-1/

English, Nick. "12 Complete Proteins Vegetarians Need to Know About," April 29, 2014.
http://greatist.com/health/complete-vegetarian-proteins

Environmental Working Group. "EWG's Shopper's Guide to Pesticides in Produce," April 1 2014.
http://www.ewg.org/foodnews/summary.php

Essence-of-Life.com. "A List of Acid/Alkaline Forming Foods," retrieved on October 1, 2014.
http://www.rense.com/1.mpicons/acidalka.htm

Guthrie, Catherine. "Fertility Diet: The Nutrients You Need to Conceive," retrieved on July 15, 2014.
http://www.babycenter.com/0_fertility-diet-the-nutrients-you-need-to-conceive_1460692.bc?showAll=true

Haas, Elson. *Staying Healthy with Nutrition: The Complete Guide to Diet and Nutritional Medicine*. Berkeley, CA: Celestial Arts, 2006.

Hanuise, Pauline. "How to Support and Detox Your Kidneys," September 30, 2013.
http://www.mindbodygreen.com/0-10914/how-to-support-detox-your-kidneys.html

Harvard Health Publications. "The Truth About Vitamins and Minerals: Choosing the Nutrients You Need to Stay Healthy," retrieved on July 10, 2014.
http://www.helpguide.org/harvard/vitamins_and_minerals.htm

Go Red for Women. "Heart Statistics at a Glance," retrieved July 15, 2014.
https://www.goredforwomen.org/about-heart-disease/facts_about_heart_disease_in_women-sub-category/statistics-at-a-glance/

Ipatenco, Sara. "Carbs and Nutrition of Movie Theater Popcorn," last updated on January 30, 2014.
http://www.livestrong.com/article/284046-carbs-nutrition-of-movie-theater-popcorn/

Jamieson, Alex. *The Great American Detox Diet*. New York: Rodale, 2005.

Keele University. "Aluminum in Breast Tissue: A Possible Factor in the Cause of Breast Cancer," September 2, 2007.
http://www.sciencedaily.com/releases/2007/08/070831210302.htm

Landau, Elizabeth. "Why Are Food Allergies on the Rise?" August 3, 2010.
http://www.cnn.com/2010/HEALTH/08/03/food.allergies.er.gut/

Lynn, Michaela, and Michael Chrisemer, NC. *Baby Greens: A Live-Food Approach for Children of All Ages.* Berkeley, CA: Frog Books, 2004.

Marie, Joanne. "How Does a Poor Diet Affect Fetal Development?" retrieved on July 10, 2014.
http://livehealthy.chron.com/poor-diet-affect-fetal-development-1097.html

Morrison, Jeffrey A. *Cleanse Your Body, Clear Your Mind.* New York: Hudson Street Press, 2011.

National Center for Health Statistics. *Health, United States, 2011: With Special Feature on Socioeconomic Status and Health.* Hyattsville, MD: 2012.

National Institute of Health. "What Are Risk Factors for Preterm Labor and Birth?" last updated on March 11, 2014.
http://www.nichd.nih.gov/health/topics/preterm/conditioninfo/Pages/who_risk.aspx

Nelson, Nina. "How and Why You Should Cleanse or Detoxify Before Pregnancy," January 9, 2013.
http://modernalternativepregnancy.com/2013/01/09/how-and-why-you-should-cleanse-or-detoxify-before-pregnancy/#.U6HreK78dbI

O'Conner, Siobhan and Alexandra Spunt. *No More Dirty Looks: The Truth About Your Beauty Products and the Ultimate Guide to Safe and Clean Cosmetics.* New York: DaCapo Lifelong Press, 2010.

Ogden, CL, Carroll, MD, Kit, BK, Flegal, KM (2014). "Prevalence of Childhood and Adult Obesity in the United States, 2011–2012." *Journal of the American Medical Association.* 311(8): 806–814.

Peta. "The Natural Human Diet," November 7, 2010.
http://www.peta.org/living/food/natural-human-diet/

Picco, Michael F. "Digestion: How Long Does It Take?"
October 30, 2012.
http://www.mayoclinic.com/health/digestive-system/an00896

Planck, Nina. *Real Food for Mother and Baby: The Fertility Diet, Eating for Two, and Baby's First Foods*. New York: Bloomsbury, 2009.

Pratt, Steven. *SuperFoods Rx for Pregnancy: The Right Choices for a Healthy, Smart, Super Baby*. Hoboken, NJ: John Wiley & Sons, 2013.

Reece, Tamekia. "10 Ways He Can Have Better Babymaking Sperm," retrieved on July 12, 2014.
http://www.parents.com/getting-pregnant/trying-to-conceive/tips/better-babymaking-sperm-healthy/

Rose, Natalia. *Raw Food Life Energy Force*. New York: Harper Collins Publishing, 2007.

Snyder, Kimberly. *The Beauty Detox Solution*. Don Mills, Ontario: Harlequin, 2011.

Walton, Alice G. "How Much Sugar Are Americans Eating?"
August 30, 2012.
http://www.forbes.com/sites/alicegwalton/2012/08/30/how-much-sugar-are-americans-eating-infographic/?&_suid=1403635189604034266615146771073

Women's Health and Fitness. "10 New 'Super Foods' for 2014," retrieved on July 20, 2014.
http://www.womenshealthandfitness.com.au/diet-nutrition/healthy-eating/1211-10-new-superfoods-for-2014?showall=&start=1

Index

Acknowledgments

I want to first and foremost thank my husband, Alex, for making me realize it's okay to show all parts of myself (even the ugly ones—can't take back seeing that birth now, can you?); my daughter, Sophie, who challenges and amazes me each and every day; my "mama" friends who have been there from the start: Lauren, Nikki, Alejandra, Adriana, April, Helena, and everyone else who has given me help through pregnancy, birth, and beyond. Life as a mother has changed me in innumerable ways. It has given me a new lens with which to view life.

Thank you to the entire team at Ulysses Press for allowing me to talk about such an important subject and to do it in my own way. To my editor, Renee Rutledge, who made stylistic choices to better the book and my writing—thank you.

Thank you to Johnny Cooke (aka "master of the universe") for encouraging me to start a different conversation. I continue to learn from you, both professionally and mentally. Thank you to my intern, Meredith Rodefer, for the research, the time, and allowing me to start sentences with: "Oh, my *intern* is looking into that..." You are magical.

And lastly, thank you to my parents for raising a child who was always enamored by food, who put it above almost anything else in her life and would literally turn into a world-class a**hole if she became tired *and* hungry. Thank you for teaching me to use my body as well as my mind, and that being strong, smart, hungry, and athletic *is* beautiful. Thank you for allowing me to realize the medicinal powers of food and how to cure almost any ailment with what's in the fridge.

About the Author

Rea Frey is an award-winning author, nutrition specialist, and International Sports Sciences Association certified trainer. She is the author of *Power Vegan: Plant-Fueled Nutrition for Maximum Health and Fitness* and *The Cheat Sheet: A Clue-by-Clue Guide to Finding Out If He's Unfaithful.* She lives in Nashville with her husband and daughter. To learn more, visit Rea's website: reafrey.com.